INSTANT REFERENCE

MEDICINE

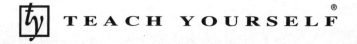

ty   TEACH YOURSELF®

For UK orders: please contact Bookpoint Ltd., 130 Milton Park, Abingdon, Oxon OX14 4SB. Telephone: (44) 01235 827720. Fax: (44) 01235 400454. Lines are open from 09.00–18.00, Monday to Saturday, with a 24-hour message answering service. E:mail address: orders@bookpoint.co.uk

For U.S.A. order enquiries: please contact McGraw-Hill Customer Services, P.O. Box 545, Blacklick, OH 43004-0545, U.S.A. Telephone: 1-800-722-4726. Fax: 1-614-755-5645.

For Canada order enquiries: please contact McGraw-Hill Ryerson Ltd., 300 Water St, Whitby, Ontario L1N 9B6, Canada. Telephone: 905 430 5000. Fax: 905 430 5020.

Long renowned as the authoritative source for self-guided learning – with more than 30 million copies sold worldwide – the *Teach Yourself* series includes over 300 titles in the fields of languages, crafts, hobbies, business and education.

British Library Cataloguing in Publication Data
A catalogue record for this title is available from The British Library.

Library of Congress Catalog Card Number: On file

First published in UK 2001 by Hodder Headline Plc., 338 Euston Road, London, NW1 3BH.

First published in US 2001 by Contemporary Books, A Division of The McGraw-Hill Companies, 4255 West Touhy Avenue, Lincolnwood (Chicago), Illinois 60712-1975 U.S.A.

The 'Teach Yourself' name and logo are registered trade marks of Hodder & Stoughton Ltd.

Picture Credits:
With special thanks to AKG:
2, 73, 75, 83, 89, 102, 105, 110, 119, 141, 164

Text Editor: Paulette Pratt
Typeset by TechType, Abingdon, Oxon
Printed in Great Britain for Hodder & Stoughton Educational, a division of Hodder Headline Plc, 338 Euston Road, London NW1 3BH by Cox & Wyman Ltd., Reading, Berkshire.

Impression number	10 9 8 7 6 5 4 3 2 1						
Year	2007	2006	2005	2004	2003	2002	2001

Contents

Bold type in the text indicates a cross reference. A plural, or possessive, is given as the cross reference, i.e. is in bold type, even if the entry to which it refers is singular.

abscess
Collection of **pus** forming in response to infection. Its presence is signalled by pain and **inflammation**. The infection causes tissue destruction in a circumscribed area and leucocytes (**white blood cells**) aggregate, forming pus. Healing occurs in most instances, with absorption of the cellular debris, but occasionally the abscess may discharge onto the skin surface. Most abscesses are due to bacterial infection. Abscesses may occur in any part of the body, in any organ. The **bacteria** are usually susceptible to **antibiotics**, but their action depends on an adequate blood supply to the site of inflammation. Thus the drugs will not reach a large abscess, which has no blood supply, and surgical drainage may be required. In pulmonary **tuberculosis** (TB), an abscess forms in the lung.

Achilles tendon
Tendon at the back of the ankle attaching the calf muscles to the heel bone. It is one of the largest tendons in the human body and can resist great tensional strain, but is sometimes torn due to excessive stress.

Ancient surgeons regarded wounds in the Achilles tendon as fatal, probably because of the Greek legend that relates how the mother of the hero Achilles dipped him, as an infant, into the River Styx so that he became invulnerable except for the heel by which she held him.

acne
Skin eruption, mainly occurring among adolescents and young adults, caused by **inflammation** of the sebaceous glands, which secrete an oily substance (sebum), the natural lubricant of the skin. Sometimes the openings of the glands become blocked, causing the formation of **pus**-filled swellings. Teenage acne is seen mainly on the face, back, and chest. There are other, less common types of

acne, sometimes caused by contact with irritant chemicals (chlo-racne). Increased hormonal activity around the onset of **puberty** stimulates the sebaceous glands to produce excessive amounts of sebum, a condition called seborrhoea. In acne, the chemical com-position of sebum may be altered by the action of **bacteria**. The changed sebum, a potent skin irritant, escapes into the surrounding dermis (the deeper layers of the skin), causing papules (hard pim-ples) or pustules (pus-containing pimples). In severe cases nodules and cysts occur and the skin may be permanently scarred. The plug blocking the outflow of sebum is a melanin-tipped core of horny material, which causes either a blackhead or a whitehead on the skin surface. Topical application of creams is useful in mild cases of acne. In other cases, **antibiotics** may be needed.

acupressure

In **alternative medicine**, generic term covering several massage techniques, mostly Chinese in origin, in which fingertip pres-sure is applied to predetermined points on the body thought to stimulate the vital energy in cor-responding organs. These techniques include **shiatsu**, developed in Japan from Chinese origins. Acupressure may be used for immediate relief of symptoms, for the maintenance of general health, and in support-ing other forms of treatment. It lends itself to application as a self-help technique.

acupuncture

In **alternative medicine**, a sys-tem based on the insertion of long, thin metal needles into

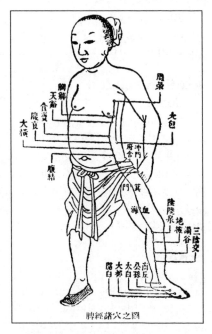

acupuncture *A Chinese diagram showing acupuncture points on the human body.*

the body at predetermined points, believed to relieve pain, to provide anaesthesia for surgery, and to assist healing. Once inserted by the practitioner, the needles are rotated manually or electrically. The method, developed in ancient China and increasingly popular in the West, is thought to work by stimulating the brain's own painkillers, the endorphins. Acupuncture is based on a theory of physiology that posits a network of life-energy pathways, or 'meridians', in the human body and some 800 'acupuncture points' where metal needles may be inserted to affect the energy flow for purposes of preventative or remedial therapy or to produce a local anaesthetic effect. Numerous studies and surveys have attested the efficacy of the method, which is widely conceded by orthodox practitioners despite the lack of an acceptable scientific explanation.

adrenaline

Or epinephrine, a **hormone** secreted by the medulla (innermost part) of the adrenal glands. Adrenaline is synthesized from a closely related substance, noradrenaline, and the two hormones are released into the bloodstream in situations of emotional or physiological stress, the so-called 'fight or flight' response. Adrenaline's action on the **liver** raises blood-sugar levels by stimulating glucose production. It also increases the **heartbeat** rate, increases blood flow to the **muscles**, reduces blood flow to the **skin** with the production of sweat, increases the rate and depth of breathing, and dilates the pupils of the eyes. Adrenaline and noradrenaline can be synthesized in the laboratory. Adrenaline is used to relieve bronchial asthma or to minimize blood loss during surgery. Noradrenaline serves to raise **blood pressure** in the treatment of shock. Adrenaline and noradrenaline have largely been replaced in therapy by synthetic drugs with milder side effects.

adverse drug reaction (ADR)

Unwanted and unexpected response to any therapeutic agent, including drugs, contrast media (used to give improved definition of bodily structures on X-rays), **intrauterine devices** (IUDs), and materials used in surgery.

afterbirth
In childbirth, the **placenta**, **umbilical cord**, and ruptured membranes, which become detached from the **uterus** and expelled from the mother's body soon after the baby's birth.

ageing
In common usage, the process of deterioration of the physical condition that eventually leads to death; in biological terms, the entire life process.

agoraphobia
Phobia involving fear of open spaces and public places. The **anxiety** produced can be so severe that some sufferers are unable to leave their homes for many years.

AIDS
Acronym for acquired immune deficiency syndrome, the gravest of the **sexually transmitted diseases** (STDs). It is caused by the human immunodeficiency **virus** (HIV), first identified in 1983. HIV is transmitted in body fluids, mainly blood and genital excretions. Infection with HIV is not synonymous with having AIDS; many people who have the virus in their blood remain well. In those who become ill the virus devastates the immune system, leaving the victim susceptible to infections and **cancers** that would not otherwise develop. In fact diagnosis of AIDS is based on the appearance of rare tumours or opportunistic infections in unexpected candidates. *Pneumocystis carinii* pneumonia, normally seen only in the malnourished or those whose immune systems have been deliberately suppressed, is common among AIDS victims and, for them, a leading cause of death. In the West the time-lag between infection with HIV and the onset of AIDS seems to be about ten years;

According to a World Health Organization (WHO) report released in May 1999, AIDS is the world's most deadly infectious disease, killing some 2.5 million people each year worldwide, 2 million of whom are in Africa.

progression is more rapid in developing countries. Today there is no cure as such but aggressive treatment with combinations of drugs can keep HIV-positive people healthy or prolong life. However, these treatments, which are expensive and complicated to administer, are not available to the overwhelming majority of HIV-infected people, most of whom live in sub-Saharan Africa.

alcoholism
Dependence on alcohol. It is characterized as an illness when consumption of alcohol interferes with normal physical or emotional health. Excessive alcohol consumption, whether through sustained ingestion or irregular drinking bouts or binges, may produce physical and psychological addiction and lead to nutritional and emotional disorders. Long-term heavy consumption of alcohol leads to diseases of the **heart**, **liver**, and peripheral nerves. Symptoms of chronic alcoholism include attacks of **delirium** tremens (DTs). Successful treatment of alcoholism depends on the motivation and cooperation of the patient. Patients accustomed to a large daily intake of alcohol may respond only to inpatient treatment where withdrawal symptoms are prevented or diminished by the administration of tranquillizing drugs. Milder cases of addictive alcoholism are treated by reinforcing the patient's desire to give up alcohol. Drugs, such as disulfiram, are regularly taken by the patient. Alcohol, even in small quantities, taken in association with disulfiram causes the patient to feel acutely ill. The drug is continued regularly until the craving for alcohol recedes. In other cases, 'aversion therapy' may be used to condition the patient to associate alcohol with unpleasant experiences (electric shocks are sometimes administered). In 'group therapy', individual willpower is strengthened by the collective motivation of the group. The principle is

❝ An alcoholic is someone you don't like who drinks as much as you do. ❞

Dylan Thomas, poet, quoted in *Dictionary of 20th Century Quotations.*

used by the voluntary society Alcoholics Anonymous, some of whose members have cured themselves and are committed to helping others.

Alexander technique
In **alternative medicine**, a method of correcting bad habits of posture, breathing, and muscular tension, which Australian therapist F M Alexander maintained cause many ailments. The technique is used to promote general health and relaxation and enhance vitality. Back troubles, **migraine**, asthma, **hypertension**, and some gastric and gynaecological disorders are among the conditions said to be alleviated by the technique, which is also thought to be effective in the prevention of disorders, particularly those of later life.

allergy
Special sensitivity of the body that makes it react with an exaggerated response of the natural immune defence mechanism to the introduction of an otherwise harmless foreign substance (allergen). Allergic symptoms are caused by the release of active substances from cells, including histamine, serotonin, and bradykinin. An extreme allergic reacion may result in low **blood pressure** and unconsciousness; this is called anaphylactic **shock**. **Hay fever** in summer is caused by an allergy to one or more kinds of pollen. Many asthmatics are allergic to certain kinds of dust or to **micro-organisms** in animal fur or feathers. There are many different kinds of allergies, producing a range of effects. Some people experience skin reactions, such as dermatitis, from drugs, cosmetics, or household cleaners; some suffer gastric upsets due to allergens in food. Various drugs can be used to counteract allergic symptoms, including **antihistamines** and steroids.

alternative medicine
Forms of medical treatment that do not use synthetic drugs or surgery in response to the symptoms of a disease but aim to treat the patient as a whole (holism, see **holistic medicine**). The emphasis is on maintaining health (with diet and exercise) and on dealing with the underlying causes rather than just the symptoms of illness. It may involve the use of herbal remedies and techniques like **acupuncture**,

homeopathy, and **chiropractic**. Some alternative treatments are increasingly accepted by orthodox medicine, but the absence of enforceable standards in some fields has led to the proliferation of eccentric or untrained practitioners.

Alzheimer's disease

The commonest manifestation of dementia, thought to afflict one in 20 people over 65. After heart disease, **cancer**, and **stroke** it is the most common cause of death in the Western world. Attacking the brain's 'grey matter', it is a disease of mental processes rather than physical function, characterized by memory loss and progressive intellectual impairment. It was first described by Alois Alzheimer in 1906. Various factors have been

In December 1999, after successful animal trials, a US trial was approved to ascertain whether gene therapy can be used to slow the development of Alzheimer's disease.

implicated in causing Alzheimer's disease, including high levels of aluminium in drinking water, infection, vitamin deficiency, brain injury, and the presence in the brain of abnormal protein deposits. The disease is known to run in families and is associated with several different gene abnormalities. While no cure is available, drug treatment early in the course of the disease may be helpful in slowing its progression.

amnesia

Loss or impairment of memory. As a clinical condition it may be caused by disease or injury to the brain, by some drugs, or by shock; in some cases it may be a symptom of an emotional disorder.

amniocentesis

Sampling of the amniotic fluid surrounding a **fetus** in the womb for diagnostic purposes. It is used to detect **Down's syndrome** and other genetic abnormalities. The procedure carries a small risk of **miscarriage**. A needle is inserted into the mother's abdominal wall and, usually under ultrasound guidance, a small amount of the amniotic fluid surrounding the fetus is withdrawn into a syringe.

This fluid, containing shed fetal cells, is sent for tests. In the laboratory, fetal cells can be cultured to provide a chromosomal profile of the unborn child (fetal karyotype), revealing any abnormality.

Amniocentesis is undertaken, usually at about the 16th week of pregnancy, to screen for a growing number of conditions, such as **spina bifida**, which may result in severe disability. The test is recommended for all high-risk mothers, including those over 35 years of age (who are at greater risk of having a Down's syndrome baby), and those with a family history of genetic abnormality.

amphetamine

Or speed, a powerful synthetic stimulant. Benzedrine was the earliest amphetamine marketed, used as a 'pep pill' in World War II to help soldiers overcome fatigue, and until the 1970s amphetamines were prescribed by doctors as an appetite suppressant for weight loss; as an antidepressant, to induce euphoria; and as a stimulant, to increase alertness. Indications for amphetamine use today are very restricted because of severe side effects, including addiction.

anabolic steroid

Any hormone of the steroid group that stimulates tissue growth. Its use in medicine is limited to the treatment of some **anaemias** and breast cancers; it may help to break up blood clots. Side effects include aggressive behaviour, masculinization in women, and reduced height in children. It is used in sports, such as weightlifting and athletics, to increase muscle bulk for greater strength and stamina, but it is widely condemned because of the side effects. In 1988 the Canadian sprinter Ben Johnson was stripped of an Olympic gold medal for having taken anabolic steroids.

anaemia

Condition caused by a shortage of **haemoglobin**, the oxygen-carrying component of **red blood cells**. The main symptoms are fatigue, pallor, breathlessness, **palpitations**, and poor resistance to infection. Treatment depends on the cause. Anaemia arises either from abnormal loss of or defective production of haemoglobin. Excessive loss occurs, for instance, with chronic slow bleeding or with accelerated destruction (haemolysis) of red blood cells. Defective production may be due to iron deficiency, vitamin B12 deficiency (pernicious anaemia), certain blood diseases (**sickle-cell disease**, thalassaemia), chronic infection, kidney disease, or certain kinds of poisoning. Untreated anaemia taxes the heart and may prove fatal.

anaesthetic
Drug that produces anaesthesia, an absence of sensation in all or part of the body. Anaesthetics are used to enable surgery without pain. Anaesthesia can also arise as a result of disease or injury of nerves. Anaesthetic agents fall into two broad categories: general or local.
- A general anaesthetic produces unconsciousness, a state of controlled coma.
- The patient undergoing local anaesthesia remains conscious but the operative site is numbed.

Where general anaesthesia is planned, pre-medication is given to reduce anxiety and dry up bronchial secretions which could be inhaled during surgery. Anaesthesia is usually induced with an intravenous drug but an inhalational agent (gas), or a combination of the two, may then be used. A muscle relaxant agent may be injected to facilitate surgery without the need for deeper anaesthesia; the patient's breathing is taken over by a ventilator. Local anaesthetics, which block the transmission of pain signals to the **brain**, may be applied to the surface of the body (surface or topical anaesthesia) or injected around nerves (regional anaesthesia). Regional anaesthesia is used for many procedures, including surgery on the beating heart. There are a

SAFETY OF ANAESTHESIA

Although the science of anaesthetics is 150 years old, it is only comparatively recently that safe doses have begun to be calculated correctly. It is said that when the Japanese bombed Pearl Harbour in 1941, more US servicemen were killed by anaesthetics than by bombs.

number of techniques, including nerve blocks to numb a limb and spinal anaesthesia, where the drug is injected into the spaces surrounding the **spinal cord** to deaden sensation in the lower part of the body. The most commonly used spinal technique, epidural block, is invaluable in obstetrics.

❝ Dr Snow gave that blessed Chloroform & the effect was soothing, quieting, & delightful beyond measure. ❞

Queen Victoria, describing her labour, *Journals*.

---

analgesic
Agent for relieving pain. Opiates alter the perception or appreciation of pain and are effective in controlling 'deep' visceral (internal) pain. Non opiates, such as **aspirin**, **paracetamol**, and **NSAIDs** (nonsteroidal anti-inflammatory drugs), relieve musculoskeletal pain and reduce inflammation in soft tissues. Pain is felt when electrical stimuli travel along a nerve pathway, from peripheral nerve fibres to the brain via the **spinal cord**. Temporary or permanent analgesia may be achieved by injection of an anaesthetic agent into, or the severing of, a nerve. Implanted devices enable patients to deliver controlled electrical stimulation to block pain impulses. Production of the body's natural opiates, endorphins, can be manipulated by techniques such as relaxation and biofeedback. However, for the severe pain of, for example, terminal cancer, opiate analgesics are required.

aneurysm
Weakening in the wall of an artery, causing it to balloon outwards with the risk of rupture and serious, often fatal, blood loss. If detected in time, some accessible aneurysms can be repaired.

Aortic aneurysms ensue mostly from **arteriosclerosis** and the risks are heightened by high blood pressure and smoking. Other causes include diseases of the blood vessels, hereditary connective tissue disorders, and physical **trauma**. Most aneurysms within the brain are congenital. They may rupture, causing bleeding into the brain tissue.

angina

Or angina pectoris, is severe pain in the chest due to impaired blood supply to the heart muscle because a coronary artery is narrowed. Faintness and difficulty in breathing accompany the pain. Treatment is by drugs or surgery.

anorexia

Lack of desire to eat, or refusal to eat, especially the pathological condition of anorexia nervosa, most often found in adolescent girls and young women who may be obsessed with the desire to lose weight but it can also affect older women and males. Compulsive eating, or **bulimia**, distortions of body image, and depression often accompany anorexia. Anorexia nervosa may be mild and transient or severe and chronic. The condition is characterized by severe self-imposed restriction of food intake, leading to serious, often life-threatening weight loss. Over time, every organ in the body may be adversely affected and female anorexics may cease to menstruate. Weakness and debility may be exacerbated by attempts to purge, including forced vomiting and the inappropriate use of **laxatives** and **diuretics**. In extreme cases there is a risk of sudden death from heart failure. Treatment involves measures to restore body weight together with psychotherapy and sometimes drug therapy. In view of the very real risk of death, estimates vary between 10 and 20 per cent, many experts feel that feeding an anorexic patient by artificial means is justified. The causes of anorexia nervosa are not fully understood. However, since it is overwhelmingly a disorder of affluent nations, there is a clear association with social pressures, including dysfunctional family dynamics and the Western preoccupation with thinness.

antibiotic

Drug that kills or inhibits the growth of **bacteria** and fungi. It is derived from living organisms such as fungi or bacteria, which distinguishes it from synthetic antimicrobials. The earliest antibiotics, the **penicillins**, came into use from 1941 and were quickly joined by chloramphenicol, the cephalosporins, erythromycins, tetracyclines, and aminoglycosides. A range of broad-spectrum antibiotics, the 4-quinolones, was developed in 1989, of which ciprofloxacin was the first. Each class and individual antibiotic acts in a different way and may be effective against either a broad spectrum or a specific type of disease-causing agent. Use of antibiotics has become more selective as side effects, such as toxicity, **allergy**, and resistance, have become better understood. Bacteria have the ability to develop resistance following repeated or inadequate doses, so that more advanced and synthetic antibiotics are continually required to overcome them.

antibody

Protein molecule produced in the blood by lymphocytes (type of white **blood cell**) in response to the presence of foreign or invading substances (antigens); such substances include the proteins carried on the surface of infecting **micro-organisms**. Antibody production is only one aspect of immunity in vertebrates.

Each antibody acts against only one kind of antigen, combining with it to form a 'complex'. This action may render antigens harmless or it may destroy micro-organisms by setting off chemical changes that cause them to self-destruct. In other cases, the formation of a complex will cause antigens to form clumps that can then be detected and engulfed by white blood cells. Each bacterial or viral infection will bring about the manufacture of a specific antibody, which will then fight the disease. Many diseases can only be contracted once because antibodies remain in the blood after the infection has passed, preventing any further invasion. **Vaccines** boost a person's resistance by causing the production of antibodies specific to particular infections.

antidepressant

Any drug used to relieve symptoms in depressive illness. The main groups are:

- the selective serotonin-reuptake inhibitors (SSRIs)
- the tricyclic antidepressants (TCADs)
- the monoamine oxidase inhibitors (MAOIs).

They all act by altering chemicals available to the central nervous system. All may produce serious side effects.

antidote
Drug used to counteract a poison. For instance, acetylcysteine is an antidote to **paracetamol** and is administered to prevent liver damage following overdosage.

antihistamine
Any substance that counteracts the effects of histamine. Antihistamines may occur naturally or they may be synthesized. H1 antihistamines are used to relieve **allergies**, alleviating symptoms such as runny nose, itching, swelling, or asthma. H2 antihistamines suppress acid production by the stomach and are used in the treatment of peptic ulcers.

antiseptic
Any substance that kills or inhibits the growth of **micro-organisms**. The use of antiseptics was pioneered by Joseph **Lister**. He used carbolic acid (phenol), which is a weak antiseptic; antiseptics such as TCP are derived from this.

anxiety
Emotional state of fear or apprehension. It is a normal response in stressful situations but is frequently a symptom of mental disorder. Anxiety is experienced as a feeling of suspense, helplessness, or alternating hope and despair together with excessive alertness and characteristic bodily changes such as tightness in the throat, disturbances in breathing and heartbeat, sweating, and diarrhoea. In psychiatry, an anxiety state is a type of **neurosis** in which the anxiety either seems to arise for no reason or else is out of proportion to what may have caused it. 'Phobic anxiety' refers to the irrational fear that characterizes **phobia**. Abnormal anxiety is a debilitating condition which may dominate a person's life.

appendicitis
Inflammation of the appendix, a small, blind extension of the bowel

in the lower right abdomen. In an acute attack, the pus-filled appendix may burst, causing a potentially lethal spread of infection (peritonitis). Treatment is by removal (appendicectomy). **See also:** *peritoneum.*

Aristotle (384–322 BC)

Greek philosopher acknowledged as the father of biological science. The son of a physician, he was the founder of comparative anatomy and a keen naturalist. It was from animal dissections that he was able to describe and name various structures. His drawing of the male urogenital system is the earliest known anatomical diagram. Many of Aristotle's conclusions were erroneous, including his view of the brain as being merely a cooling organ for the heart, which, he believed, was the seat of life and intelligence. He also deduced that the arteries contained air, instead of blood. Nevertheless, his influence as a natural scientist pursuing methodical inquiry was considerable.

A one-time tutor of Alexander the Great, Aristotle settled in Athens in 355 BC, opening his Lyceum as a centre for study and research.

aromatherapy

In **alternative medicine**, the use of oils and essences derived from plants, flowers, and wood resins. Bactericidal properties and beneficial effects upon physiological functions are attributed to the oils, which are sometimes ingested but generally massaged into the skin. Aromatherapy was first used in ancient Greece and Egypt, but became a forgotten art until the 1930s, when a French chemist accidentally spilt lavender oil over a cut and found that the wound healed without a scar. However, it was not until the 1970s that aromatherapy began to achieve widespread popularity. By the 1990s aromatherapy had gained a degree of acceptance in mainstream health treatment in Britain and had started to become available on the National Health Service. In 1996, the Royal Liverpool University Hospital became the first in Britain to provide aromatherapy as part of a range of alternative treatments.

arteriosclerosis

Hardening of the arteries, with thickening and loss of elasticity. The term is used loosely as a synonym for **atherosclerosis**.

artery

Vessel that carries blood from the heart to the rest of the body. It is built to withstand considerable pressure, having thick walls which contain smooth muscle fibres. During contraction of the heart muscle, arteries expand in diameter to allow for the sudden increase in pressure that occurs; the resulting pulse or pressure wave can be felt at the wrist. Not all arteries carry oxygenated (oxygen-rich) blood; the pulmonary arteries convey deoxygenated (oxygen-poor) blood from the heart to the lungs. Arteries are flexible, elastic tubes consisting of three layers, the middle of which is muscular; its rhythmic contraction aids the pumping of blood around the body.

arthritis

Inflammation of the joints, with pain, swelling, and restricted motion. Many conditions may cause arthritis, including gout, infection, and trauma to the joint. There are three main forms of arthritis:

- **rheumatoid arthritis**
- osteoarthritis
- septic arthritis.

asphyxia

Suffocation; a lack of oxygen that produces a potentially lethal buildup of carbon dioxide waste in the tissues. Asphyxia may arise from any one of a number of causes, including inhalation of smoke or poisonous gases, obstruction of the windpipe, strangulation or smothering. If it is not promptly relieved, brain damage or death ensue.

aspirin

Acetylsalicylic acid, a popular analgesic developed in the late 19th century as a household remedy for aches and pains. It relieves pain and reduces **inflammation** and **fever**. It is derived from the white willow tree, *Salix alba*, and is one of the world's most widely used drugs. Regular use of aspirin is recommended for people at increased risk of **heart attack**, **thrombosis**, and some kinds of **stroke**. However, it tends to irritate the lining of the stomach and may cause bleeding. It is no longer considered suitable for children under 12 because of a link with a rare disease, Reye's syndrome. Aspirin works by inhibiting production of prostaglandins, substances which act as mediators in the inflammatory process. However, with the advent of newer, less irritant

Aspirin was refined from salicylic acid, which occurs naturally in willow bark, by the German chemist Felix Hoffman. It was first marketed in 1899.

anti-inflammatory drugs, it is now rarely used in high doses and only then under specialist supervision. Even so, aspirin continues to be hailed as a 'wonder drug' with new benefits constantly being reported, such as its ability to prevent gum disease (**periodontal disease**).

See also: *paracetamol.*

asthma

Chronic condition characterized by difficulty in **breathing** due to spasm of the bronchi (air passages) in the **lungs**. Attacks may be provoked by **allergy**, infection, and stress. The incidence of asthma may be increasing as a result of air pollution and occupational hazard. Treatment is with bronchodilators to relax the bronchial muscles and thereby ease the breathing, and in severe cases by inhaled steroids that reduce inflammation of the bronchi. Approximately 5–10% of children suffer from asthma, but about a third of these will show no symptoms after adolescence, while another 5–10% of people develop the condition as adults. Growing evidence that the immune system (see **immunity**) is involved in both forms of asthma has raised the possibility of a new approach to treatment.

Extrinsic asthma, which is triggered by exposure to irritants such as pollen and dust, is more common in children and young adults. In February 1997 Brazilian researchers reported two species of dust mite actually living on children's scalps. This explains why vacuuming of bedding sometimes fails to prevent asthma attacks. The use of antidandruff shampoo should keep numbers of mites down by reducing their food supply.

atherosclerosis
Thickening and hardening of the walls of the arteries, associated with the formation of fatty deposits (atheroma), mostly of cholesterol.

athlete's foot
Commonest type of ringworm, affecting the skin between the toes. A fungal infection, it is highly contagious. The medical name is *tinea pedis*.

autism, infantile
Rare disorder, generally present from birth, characterized by a withdrawn state and a failure to develop normal relationships. Behaviour is compulsive and ritualistic and the child fails to develop normally in language or social behaviour. The condition, which is up to four times more common in boys than girls, tends to persist throughout life. Although autistic children may, rarely, show signs of high intelligence, up to 70 per cent have some degree of mental retardation. The cause is unknown, but there may be a genetic factor involved and some autistic children and adults have brain abnormalities. Special education may bring about some improvement. Drugs are sometimes used to control disruptive symptoms. A link has been suggested between autism and the triple **MMR** vaccine. However, medical investigation has failed to substantiate the claim.

autoimmunity
In medicine, a condition where the body's immune responses (see **immunity**) are mobilized not against 'foreign' matter, such as invading germs, but against the body itself. Diseases considered to be of autoimmune origin include myasthenia gravis, **rheumatoid arthritis**, and lupus erythematous.

In autoimmune diseases T-lymphocytes reproduce to excess to home in on a target (properly a foreign disease-causing molecule); however, molecules of the body's own tissue that resemble the target may also be attacked, for example insulin-producing cells, resulting in insulin-dependent **diabetes**. If certain joint membrane cells are attacked, then rheumatoid arthritis may result; and if myelin, the basic protein of the nervous system, is attacked, then **multiple sclerosis** results.

Ayurveda

Naturopathic system of medicine widely practised in India and based on principles derived from the ancient Hindu scriptures, the Vedas. Hospital treatments and remedial prescriptions tend to be nonspecific and to coordinate holistic therapies for body, mind, and spirit.

B

Bach flower healing

A homeopathic system of medical therapy developed in the 1920s by the English physician Edward Bach. Based on the healing properties of wild flowers, it seeks to alleviate mental and emotional causes of disease rather than their physical symptoms.

bacteria

(Singular bacterium) Microscopic single-celled organisms lacking a nucleus. Bacteria are widespread, present in soil, air, and water, and as parasites on and in other living things. Some parasitic bacteria cause disease by producing **toxins** but others are harmless and may even benefit their hosts. Bacteria are classified biochemically, but their varying shapes provide a rough grouping; for example, cocci are round or oval, bacilli are rodlike, spirilla are spiral, and vibrios are shaped like commas. Bacteria belong in two broad classes (called Gram positive and negative) according to their reactions to certain stains, or dyes, used in microscopy. The staining technique, called the Gram test after Danish bacteriologist Hans Gram, allows doctors to identify many bacteria quickly. Bacteria have a large loop of **DNA**, sometimes called a bacterial chromosome. In addition there are often small, circular pieces of DNA known as plasmids that carry spare genetic information. These plasmids can readily move from one bacterium to another (plasmid transfer), even though the bacteria may be of different species. In a sense, they are

---

BACTERIAL GUESTS

Bacteria on and in the human body outnumber the number of cells that constitute the body.

parasites within the bacterial cell, but they survive by coding characteristics that promote the survival of their hosts. For example, some plasmids confer antibiotic resistance on the bacteria they inhabit.

barbiturate

Hypnosedative drug, commonly known as a sleeping pill. Most barbiturates, being highly addictive, are no longer prescribed and are listed as controlled substances. Tolerance develops quickly in the user so that increasingly large doses are required to induce sleep. A barbiturate's action persists for hours or days, causing confused, aggressive behaviour or disorientation. Overdosage causes death by inhibiting the breathing centre in the **brain**. Short-acting barbiturates are used as anaesthetics to induce general anaesthesia; slow-acting ones may be prescribed for **epilepsy**.

basal metabolic rate (BMR)

Minimum amount of energy needed by the body to maintain life. It is measured when the subject is awake but resting and includes the energy required to keep the heart beating, sustain breathing, repair tissues, and keep the brain and nerves functioning. Measuring the subject's consumption of oxygen gives an accurate value for BMR because oxygen is needed to release energy from food.

BMR varies from males to females. It is highest in children and declines with age. Disease, including mental illness, can make it rise or fall. **Hormones** from the **thyroid** gland control the BMR.

BCG

Abbreviation for bacille *Calmette-Guérin*, the bacillus injected as a **vaccine** to confer active immunity to **tuberculosis** (TB). BCG was developed by Albert Calmette and Camille Guérin in France in 1921 from live bovine TB bacilli. These **bacteria** were bred in the laboratory over many generations until they became attenuated (weakened). Each inoculation contains just enough live, attenuated bacilli to provoke an immune response: the formation of specific antibodies. The **vaccine** provides protection for 50–80% of infants vaccinated.

Bernard, Claude (1813–1878)

French physiologist and founder of experimental medicine. Bernard first demonstrated that digestion is not restricted to the stomach but takes place throughout the small intestine. He discovered the digestive input of the **pancreas**, several functions of the **liver**, and the vasomotor nerves which dilate and contract the blood vessels and thus regulate body temperature.

beta-blocker

Any of a class of drugs that block impulses that stimulate certain nerve endings (beta receptors) serving the heart muscle. This reduces the heart rate and the force of contraction, which in turn reduces the amount of oxygen (and therefore the blood supply) required by the heart. Beta-blockers may be useful in the treatment of **angina**, arrhythmia (abnormal heart rhythms), and raised **blood pressure**, and following **heart attacks**. They must be withdrawn from use gradually.

biological clock

Regular internal rhythm of activity, produced by unknown mechanisms, and not dependent on external time signals. In higher organisms, there appears to be a series of clocks of graded importance. For example, although body temperature and activity cycles are normally 'set' to 24 hours, the two cycles may vary independently, showing that two clock mechanisms are involved.

Exposure to bright light can change the biological clock and help, for example, people suffering from **jet lag** and **seasonal affective disorder (SAD)**.

biopsy

Removal of a living tissue sample from the body for diagnostic examination.

birthmark or naevus

Any mark or blemish on the skin that has been present since birth. There are many types of birthmark, including **moles**, patches of discoloration, or clusters of small blood vessels, such as the 'strawberry mark'.

bladder

Hollow, elastic-walled organ which stores the urine produced in the **kidneys**. Urine enters the bladder through two ureters, one leading from each kidney, and leaves it through the urethra.

blindness

Complete absence or impairment of sight. It may be caused by heredity, accident, disease, or deterioration with age. Age-related macular degeneration (AMD), the commonest form of blindness, occurs as the retina gradually deteriorates with age. It affects 1% of people over the age of 70, with many more experiencing marked reduction in sight. Retinitis pigmentosa, a common cause of blindness, is a hereditary disease affecting 1.2 million people worldwide.

blind spot

Area where the optic nerve and blood vessels pass through the retina of the **eye**. No visual image can be formed as there are no light-sensitive cells in this part of the retina, thus the organism is blind to objects that fall in this part of the visual field.

blister

Swelling on the surface of the body containing clear fluid (serum) or, more rarely, blood or **pus**. Blisters occur mostly on the skin of the hands or feet and are caused by friction.

blood

Fluid circulating in the arteries, veins, and capillaries. Blood carries nutrients and oxygen to each body cell and removes waste products such as carbon dioxide. It is also important in the immune response and in the distribution of heat throughout the body. Blood makes up 5% of the body weight. It is composed of a fluid called **plasma**, in which are suspended microscopic cells of three main varieties:

- **Red blood cells** (erythrocytes) form nearly half the volume of the blood, with about 6 million red cells in every millilitre of an adult's blood. They transport oxygen around the body. Their red coloration is caused by haemoglobin.
- **White blood cells** (leucocytes) are of various kinds. Some (phagocytes) ingest invading **bacteria** and so protect the body from disease; these also help to repair injured tissues. Others (lymphocytes) produce **antibodies**, which help provide immunity.
- Blood platelets (thrombocytes) assist in the clotting of blood.

Blood cells constantly wear out and die and are replaced from the bone marrow. Red blood cells die at the rate of 200 billion per day but the body produces new cells at an average rate of 9,000 million per hour. Arterial blood, which is rich in oxygen, is bright red in colour; venous blood, containing little oxygen, is dark red.

blood clotting

Complex series of events (known as the blood clotting cascade) that prevents excessive bleeding after injury. The result is the formation of a meshwork of protein fibres (fibrin) and trapped blood cells over the cut blood vessels. When platelets (cell fragments) in the bloodstream come into contact with a damaged blood vessel, they and the vessel wall itself release the enzyme thrombokinase, which brings about the conversion of the inactive enzyme prothrombin into the active thrombin. Thrombin in turn catalyzes the conversion of the soluble protein fibrinogen, present in blood **plasma**, to the insoluble fibrin. This fibrous protein forms a net over the wound that traps **red blood cells** and seals the wound; the resulting jellylike clot hardens on exposure to air to form a scab. Calcium, vitamin K, and a variety of enzymes called factors are also necessary for efficient blood clotting. **Haemophilia** is one of several diseases in which the clotting mechanism is impaired. **See also**: *thrombosis.*

blood group

Any of the types into which blood is classified according to the presence or otherwise of certain antigens on the surface of its red cells.

Red blood cells of one individual may carry molecules on their surface that act as antigens in another individual whose red blood cells lack these molecules. The two main antigens are designated A and B. These give rise to four blood groups: having A only (A), having B only (B), having both (AB), and having neither (O). Each of these groups may or may not contain the **rhesus factor**. Correct typing of blood groups is vital in transfusion, since incompatible types of donor and recipient blood will result in coagulation, with possible death of the recipient.

The ABO system was first described by Austrian scientist Karl Landsteiner in 1902. Subsequent research revealed at least 14 main types of blood group systems, 11 of which are involved with induced antibody production. Blood typing is also of importance in forensic medicine, cases of disputed paternity, and in anthropological studies.

blood poisoning

Presence in the bloodstream of quantities of **bacteria** or bacterial toxins sufficient to cause serious illness.

blood pressure

Pressure, or tension, of the blood against the inner walls of blood vessels, especially the arteries, due to the muscular pumping activity of the **heart**. Abnormally high blood pressure (**hypertension**) may be associated with various conditions or arise with no obvious cause; abnormally low blood pressure (hypotension) occurs in **shock** and after excessive fluid or blood loss from any cause.

The left ventricle of the heart pumps blood into the arterial system. This pumping is assisted by waves of muscular contraction by the arteries themselves but resisted by the elasticity of the inner and outer walls of the arteries. Pressure is greatest when the heart ventricle contracts (systole) and lowest when the ventricle relaxes (diastole). Blood pressure is measured in millimetres of mercury (the height of a column on the measuring instrument, a sphygmomanometer). Normal blood pressure varies with age, but in a young healthy adult it is around 120/80 mm Hg; the first number represents the systolic pressure and the second the diastolic. Large deviations from the normal range usually indicate ill health.

blood test
Laboratory evaluation of a blood sample. There are numerous blood tests, from simple typing to establish the **blood group** to sophisticated biochemical assays of substances, such as hormones, present in the blood only in minute quantities. The majority of tests fall into one of three categories:

- haematology (testing the state of the blood itself)
- microbiology (identifying infection)
- blood chemistry (reflecting chemical events elsewhere in the body).

Before operations, a common test is **haemoglobin** estimation to determine how well a patient might tolerate blood loss during surgery.

body temperature
Intensity of heat deep in the tissues (core temperature) as measured on a thermometer. In the healthy adult it is normally 37°C. Any significant departure from this norm is potentially serious (although fever is a necessary response to infection). Hyperthermia (temperature above 41°C) and **hypothermia** (below 35°C) are life-threatening. Body temperature is controlled by the hypothalamus in the brain. It serves as a thermostat, initiating physiological measures to lose or gain heat. Heat is conserved by constriction of the superficial blood vessels, causing the blood to flow in deeper vessels. To lose heat, the superficial blood vessels dilate and sweating occurs (evaporation).
  See also: *heatstroke.*

boil
Small pus-filled swelling originating around a hair follicle or in a sweat gland. Usually caused by local infection with *Staphylococcus aureus* bacterium, boils are most likely to form if resistance is low or diet inadequate.

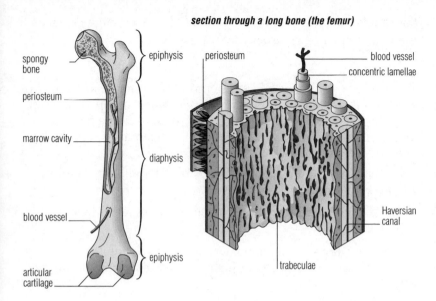

section through a long bone (the femur)

spongy bone

epiphysis

periosteum

blood vessel

concentric lamellae

periosteum

marrow cavity

diaphysis

blood vessel

epiphysis

trabeculae

Haversian canal

articular cartilage

bone *A section through the femur, or thighbone. The upper end of the femur is made up of spongy bone, which has a fine lacework structure designed to transmit the weight of the body. The shaft of the femur consists of hard compact bone designed to resist bending. Fine channels carrying blood vessels, nerves, and lymphatics interweave even the densest bone.*

bone

Hard connective tissue comprising the **skeleton**. Bone is composed of a network of collagen fibres impregnated with mineral salts (largely calcium phosphate and calcium carbonate), a combination that gives it great density and strength, comparable in some cases with that of reinforced concrete. Enclosed within this solid matrix are bone cells, blood vessels, and nerves. The interior of the long bones of the limbs consists of a spongy matrix filled with a soft marrow that produces blood cells.

brain

A mass of interconnected nerve cells forming the upper part of the **central nervous system,** whose activities it coordinates and controls. The brain is contained by the skull. At the base of the brainstem, the

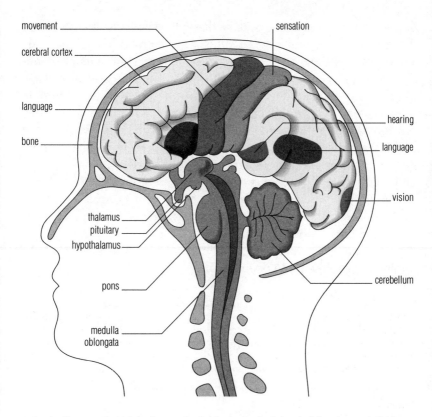

brain *The structure of the human brain. At the back of the skull lies the cerebellum, which coordinates reflex actions that control muscular activity. The medulla controls respiration, heartbeat, and blood pressure. The hypothalamus is concerned with instinctive drives and emotions. The thalamus relays signals to and from various parts of the brain. The pituitary gland controls the body's hormones. Distinct areas of the large convoluted cerebral hemispheres that fill most of the skull are linked to sensations, such as hearing and sight, and voluntary activities, such as movement.*

medulla oblongata contains centres for the control of respiration, **heartbeat** rate and strength, and **blood pressure**. Overlying this is the cerebellum, which is concerned with coordinating complex muscular activities such as maintaining posture and moving limbs. The cerebral hemispheres (cerebrum) are paired outgrowths of the front end of the forebrain, involved in the integration of all sensory input and motor output, and in thought, emotions, memory, and behaviour. Many of the nerve fibres from the two sides of the body cross over as they enter the brain, so that the left cerebral hemisphere is associated with the right side of the body and vice versa. A certain asymmetry develops in the two halves of the cerebrum. In right-handed people, the left hemisphere seems to play a greater role in controlling verbal and some mathematical skills, whereas the right hemisphere is more involved in spatial perception. In the brain, nerve impulses are passed across synapses by neurotransmitters, as in other parts of the nervous system. The cerebrum is the largest part of the brain, carrying the **cerebral cortex**. This consists of a thick surface layer of cell bodies (grey matter), below which fibre tracts (white matter) connect various parts of the cortex to each other and to other points in the central nervous system. The surface of the brain is convoluted into deep folds.

❝ BRAIN. An apparatus with which we think that we think. ❞

Ambrose Bierce, writer and journalist, *The Devils Dictionary*.

---

breathing

The muscular movements whereby air is taken into the **lungs** and then expelled, a form of gas exchange. Breathing is sometimes referred to as external respiration, for true respiration is a cellular (internal) process. In order for oxygen to be passed to the **blood** and carbon dioxide removed, air is drawn into the lungs (inhaled) by the contraction of the diaphragm and intercostal muscles; relaxation of these muscles enables air to be breathed out (exhaled). The rate of breathing is controlled by the **brain**. High levels of activity lead to a greater demand for oxygen and an increased rate of breathing.

breech presentation

Abnormal position of the baby awaiting delivery where it is lying with the buttocks nearest the birth canal rather than in the normal head-down position. It can sometimes be corrected by a manoeuvre known as cephalic version: turning the baby so that its head can be delivered first.

brittle bone disease
Rare inherited disorder in which the main feature is extreme fragility and brittleness of **bone**. The tendency to fracture sometimes diminishes after puberty. The medical name is *osteogenesis imperfecta*.

bronchitis
Inflammation of the bronchi (air passages) of the **lungs**, usually caused initially by a viral infection, such as the common **cold** or **influenza** (flu). It is aggravated by environmental pollutants, especially **smoking**, and results in a persistent cough, irritated mucus-secreting glands, and large amounts of **sputum**.

bruise or contusion
Patch of discoloration on the skin resulting from seepage of blood from damaged underlying vessels. It is caused by injury, usually a blow. The change in colour of a bruise is due to degradation of **haemoglobin** in the tissues.

BSE
Abbreviation for bovine spongiform encephalopathy ('mad cow disease'), a disease of cattle allied to scrapie in sheep. It attacks the **nervous system**, causing aggression, lack of co-ordination, and collapse. First identified in 1986, in the UK, it is thought to have given rise

❝ We are leading the world in BSE research, which is quite right because we did, after all, give the world BSE in the first place. ❞

Whitehall spokesperson, on plans for a 7-year research programme into mad cow disease, *The Independent*, 1998.

to a new variant of the human disease **CJD**. BSE is one of a group of diseases known as the transmissible spongiform encephalopathies since they are characterized by the appearance of spongy changes in brain tissue. The cause of these universally fatal diseases is not fully understood but they are associated with an abnormal protein, called a prion, which may be inborn or acquired from contaminated tissue.

bulimia

Condition of continuous, uncontrolled overeating. Considered a manifestation of stress or depression, this eating disorder is found chiefly in young women. However, it may also arise as a result of brain damage or disease. When compensated for by forced vomiting or overdoses of laxatives, the condition is called bulimia nervosa. It is sometimes associated with **anorexia.**

bunion

Inflammation of the joint between the big toe and the first metatarsal bone. It tends to displace the big toe inwards, causing a bony prominence. It is due to the wearing of ill-fitting shoes. Podiatry can remove painful callosities. Underlying foot problems may be treated with surgical shoes with a broad, deep toe.

burn

Destruction of body tissue by extremes of temperature, corrosive chemicals, electricity, or radiation. First-degree burns may cause reddening; second-degree burns cause blistering and irritation but usually heal spontaneously; third-degree burns are disfiguring and may be life-threatening. Burns cause **plasma**, the fluid component of the blood, to leak from the blood vessels, and it is this loss of circulating fluid that engenders **shock**. Emergency treatment is needed for third-degree burns in order to replace the fluid volume, prevent infection (a serious threat to the severely burned), and reduce pain. Plastic,

Artificial **skin** may be used to form lattice structures similar to dermis, enabling the patient's own skin to regenerate. It protects the burned area from loss of fluid and reduces the likelihood of infection.

or reconstructive, surgery, including skin grafting, may be required to compensate for damaged tissue and minimize disfigurement. If a skin graft is necessary, dead tissue must be removed from a burn (a process known as debridement) so that the patient's blood supply can nourish the graft.

Caesarean section

Surgical operation to deliver a baby by way of an incision in the mother's abdominal and uterine walls. It may be recommended for almost any obstetric complication implying a threat to mother or baby.

callus

Growth of healing tissue, also containing blood and bone-forming cells, that forms around the ends of a **bone** following a fracture. Callus formation is an important factor in the union of the fracture.

cancer

Group of diseases characterized by abnormal proliferation of cells. Cancerous (malignant) cells are usually degenerate, capable only of reproducing themselves (tumour formation). Malignant cells tend to spread from their site of origin by travelling through the bloodstream or lymphatic system (see **metastasis**). Cancer kills about 6 million people a year worldwide.

There are more than 100 types of cancer. Some, like lung or bowel cancer, are common; others are rare. The likely causes remain unexplained. Triggering agents (**carcinogens**) include chemicals such as those found in cigarette smoke, other forms of smoke, asbestos dust, exhaust fumes, and many industrial chemicals. Some viruses can also trigger the cancerous growth of cells, as can X-rays and exposure to other forms of ionizing radiation. Dietary factors are important in some cancers; for example, lack of fibre in the diet may predispose people to bowel cancer and a diet high in animal fats and low in fresh vegetables and fruit increases the risk of breast cancer. Psychological stress may increase the risk of cancer.

Cancer is by no means incurable, particularly in the case of certain tumours, including **Hodgkin's disease**, acute **leukaemia**, and testicular cancer. Cures are sometimes achieved with specialized treatments, such as surgery, **chemotherapy**, and irradiation, or a combination of all three. Public health programmes are concerned with prevention and early detection.

❝ While there are several chronic diseases more destructive to life than cancer, none is more feared. ❞

Charles H Mayo, physician, *Annals of Surgery* (1926).

---

carbohydrate

A chemical compound composed of carbon, hydrogen, and oxygen with the basic formula $C_m(H_2O)_n$ and some related compounds. In the form of sugars and starches, carbohydrates are an important part of a balanced diet, providing energy for life processes including growth and movement. Excess carbohydrate intake can be converted into **fat** and stored in the body. The simplest carbohydrates are sugars (monosaccharides, such as glucose and fructose, and disaccharides, such as sucrose), which are soluble compounds, some with a sweet taste. When these basic sugar units are joined together in long chains or branching structures they form polysaccharides, such as starch and glycogen, which serve as food stores.

carcinogen

Any agent that increases the chance of a cell becoming cancerous (see **cancer**), including various chemical compounds, some viruses, X-rays, and other forms of ionizing radiation. The term is often used more narrowly to mean chemical carcinogens only.

cardiac arrest

Sudden failure of the pumping action of the heart. The victim loses consciousness and stops breathing. Without **resuscitation**, death follows within a few minutes. Most hospitals have cardiac arrest teams, specially trained in cardiopulmonary resuscitation and capable of an immediate response. If **breathing** and **heartbeat** are not restarted within three minutes, the brain is irreversibly damaged.

carpal tunnel syndrome
Compression of the median nerve at the wrist. It causes pain and numbness in the index and middle fingers and weakness in the thumb. It may require surgery. Women have a higher incidence of carpal tunnel syndrome, especially those who are pregnant or who have diabetes or an under-active **thyroid** gland.

Carrel, Alexis (1873–1944)
French-born US surgeon whose experiments paved the way for organ transplantation. Working at the Rockefeller Institute, Carrel devised a way of joining blood vessels end to end (anastomosing). This was important in the development of **transplant** surgery, as was his work on keeping organs viable outside the body.

cartilage
Flexible bluish-white connective tissue made up of the protein collagen. It forms the greater part of the embryonic skeleton and is replaced by bone in the course of development, except in areas of wear such as bone endings and the discs between the backbones. It also forms structural tissue in the larynx, nose, and external ear.

cataract
Eye disease in which the crystalline lens or its capsule becomes cloudy, causing blindness. Fluid accumulates between the fibres of the lens and gives place to deposits of albumin. These coalesce into rounded bodies, the lens fibres break down, and areas of the lens or the lens capsule become filled with opaque products of degeneration. The condition nearly always affects both eyes, usually one more than the other. In most cases, the treatment is replacement of the opaque lens with an artificial implant.

catarrh
Inflammation of any **mucous membrane**, especially of the nose and throat, with increased production of **mucus**.

CAT scan or CT scan
Acronym for computerized axial tomography, a sophisticated method of **X-ray** imaging. Quick and noninvasive, CAT scanning is used as an aid to diagnosis, helping to pinpoint problems without the need for exploratory surgery. The CAT scanner passes a narrow fan of X-rays through successive slices of the suspect body part. These slices are picked up by crystal detectors in a scintillator and converted electronically into cross-sectional images displayed on a viewing screen. Gradually, using views taken from various angles, a three-dimensional picture of the organ or tissue can be assembled and irregularities analyzed.

cell
In biology, the basic structural unit of life. The human body consists of billions of cells, all adapted to carry out specific functions and organized into tissues and organs. Although these cells may differ widely in size, appearance, and function, their essential features are similar. The cytoplasm of cells contains ribosomes, which carry out protein synthesis, and **DNA**, the coded instructions for the behaviour and reproduction of the cell, which is contained within a nucleus. The only cells in the body which have no nucleus are the **red blood cells**. New cells are produced

About 3 billion cells are replaced every minute. The life span of cells varies – for example, **white blood cells** live for about 13 days, red blood cells for about 120 days, and liver cells live about 18 months. **Nerve cells** can live for a century.

from existing cells. They reproduce by division (mitosis), with each cell dividing to produce two new cells. Simple cell division, or asexual reproduction, normally results in the production of two identical daughter cells, each containing a set of chromosomes identical with those of the parent cell.

Sexual reproduction requires the production of male and female germ cells (**sperm** and ova or eggs) by a process called meiosis. During this process a cell divides twice, but its **chromosomes** are duplicated only once. Thus, four germ cells are produced, each containing half the normal number of chromosomes. In males the germ cells develop into sperm; in the female they develop into eggs. A sperm and an egg then unite (**fertilization**) to form a new cell, a zygote, which has a complete set of chromosomes, having received half its genetic information from each parent.

See also: *gene, ovary.*

central nervous system (CNS)

The **brain** and **spinal cord**, as distinct from other components of the **nervous system**. The CNS integrates all nervous function.

cerebral cortex or grey matter

Fissured outer layer of the cerebrum. Some 3 mm thick in the adult, it is the most sophisticated part of the **brain**, responsible for all higher functions and for initiating voluntary movement. Anatomists divide it into four lobes, named after the skull plates beneath which they lie: frontal, parietal, temporal, and occipital.

cervix

(Latin 'neck') Abbreviation for cervix uteri, the neck of the womb; see **uterus**.

chemotherapy

Any medical treatment with chemicals. It usually refers to treatment of cancer with cytotoxic and other drugs. The term was coined by the German bacteriologist Paul **Ehrlich** for the use of synthetic chemicals against infectious diseases.

chickenpox or varicella

Common, usually mild disease, caused by a virus of the **herpes** group and transmitted by airborne droplets. Chickenpox chiefly attacks children under the age of ten. The incubation period is two to three weeks. The temperature rises and spots (later inflamed **blisters**) develop on the trunk, then on the face and limbs. The sufferer

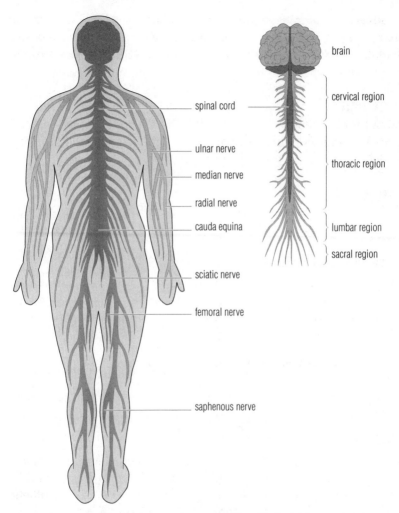

central nervous system *The central nervous system (CNS) with its associated nerves. The CNS controls and integrates body functions. In humans and other vertebrates it consists of a brain and a spinal cord, which are linked to the body's muscles and organs by means of the peripheral nervous system.*

recovers within a week but remains infectious until the last scab disappears. One attack normally gives immunity for life. However, the **virus** remains dormant in the body, sometimes becoming reactivated as **shingles** in later life.

Chickenpox can prove severe and sometimes fatal in the elderly or in people of any age with impaired **immune systems**. Vaccination is normally reserved for those at special risk from the disease.

chilblain

Painful inflammation of the skin of the feet, hands, or ears, due to cold. The affected parts turn red, swell, itch violently, and are very tender. In bad cases, the skin cracks, blisters, or ulcerates.

childbirth

The expulsion of a baby from its mother's body following pregnancy. In a broader sense, it is the period of time involving labour and delivery of the baby.

See also: *afterbirth.*

❛If men had to have babies they would only ever have one each.❜

Diana, Princess of Wales, *The Observer*, 29 July 1984.

Chinese medicine

A system based on the theory of energy currents in the body associated with the physical organs. There are a number of pathways, called meridians, along which energy is considered to flow. Each organ, or

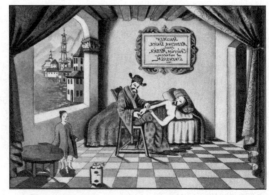

Chinese medicine *17th-century artwork depicting a Chinese doctor taking the pulse of a sick man.*

group of organs, has its own meridian and each has a number of associations — for example, one of the five Chinese elements, as well as a time of day, so that if a person is restless or depleted at a particular time daily, the site of the organic imbalance is more readily identified. Vitality is identified as chi (pronounced 'kee'); and promotion of the regular and vigorous flow of chi in the body is the object of medical practice. Many physical factors are taken into account in diagnosis, including four distinct pulses on each wrist and colour of tongue. Chinese physicians use **acupuncture** and related massage techniques (see **acupressure**) to stimulate the energy of the meridians as well as a vast assortment of herbs.

chiropody
Specialized care and treatment of the feet; practitioners are called chiropodists or podiatrists.

chiropractic
In **alternative medicine**, technique of manipulation of the spine and other parts of the body, based on the principle that physical disorders are attributable to aberrations in the functioning of the **nervous system** which are amenable to correction. Developed in the 1890s by US practitioner Daniel David Palmer, chiropractic is widely practised today by accredited therapists.

cholera
Disease caused by infection with various strains of the bacillus *Vibrio cholera,* transmitted in contaminated water and characterized by violent **diarrhoea** and vomiting. It is prevalent in many tropical areas. The formerly high death rate during epidemics has been much reduced by treatments to prevent dehydration

The sequencing of the complete cholera genome was completed in August 2000, revealing that many of the genes that enable cholera to attack humans are found on a single chromosome. The discovery should aid the development of a more effective vaccine and other drugs to combat the disease.

and loss of body salts, together with the use of antibiotics. There is an effective **vaccine** that must be repeated at frequent intervals for people exposed to continuous risk of infection. The worst epidemic in the Western hemisphere for 70 years occurred in Peru in 1991, with 55,000 confirmed cases and 258 deaths. It was believed to have been spread by the consumption of seafood contaminated by untreated sewage. 1991 was also the worst year on record for cholera in Africa with 13,000 deaths.

cholesterol
White, crystalline sterol found throughout the body, especially in **fats**, **blood**, nerve tissue, and bile; it is also provided in the diet by foods such as eggs, meat, and butter. A high level of cholesterol in the blood is thought to contribute to **atherosclerosis** (hardening of the arteries). Cholesterol is an integral part of all **cell** membranes and the starting point for steroid **hormones**, including the sex hormones. It is broken down by the **liver** into bile salts, which are involved in fat absorption in the digestive system, and it is an essential component of lipoproteins, which transport fats and fatty acids in the blood. Low-density lipoprotein cholesterol (LDL-cholesterol), when present in excess, can enter the tissues and become deposited on the surface of the arteries, causing atherosclerosis. High-density lipoprotein cholesterol (HDL-cholesterol) acts as a scavenger, transporting fat and cholesterol from the tissues to the liver to be broken down. Blood cholesterol levels can be lowered by reducing the amount of alcohol and fat in the diet and by substituting polyunsaturated fats.

chorionic villus sampling (CVS)
Biopsy of a small sample of placental tissue, carried out in early pregnancy at 10-12 weeks' gestation. Since the **placenta** forms from embryonic cells, the tissue obtained can be tested to reveal genetic abnormality in the **fetus**. The advantage of CVS over **amniocentesis** is that it provides an earlier diagnosis, so that if any abnormality is discovered, and the parents opt for an abortion, it can be carried out more safely.

chromosome

Structure in a **cell** nucleus that carries the **genes**. Each chromosome consists of one very long strand of **DNA**, coiled and folded to produce a compact body. The point on a chromosome where a particular gene occurs is known as its locus. Most higher organisms have two copies of each chromosome (diploid) but some have only one (haploid). There are 46 chromosomes in a normal human cell. Chromosomes are only visible during cell division.

XY

chromosome *The 23 pairs of chromosomes of a normal human male.*

cilia

(Singular cilium) Small hair-like organs on the surface of some cells, particularly the cells lining the upper respiratory tract. Their wavelike movements waft particles of dust and debris towards the exterior.

circumcision

Surgical removal of all or part of the foreskin (prepuce) of the **penis**, usually performed on the newborn male; it is practised especially among Jews and Muslims. Female circumcision or clitoridectomy (removal of the labia minora and/or clitoris) is practised on adolescents as well as babies in some societies in Africa and the Middle East; it is illegal in the West.

Male circumcision is mainly carried out for cultural reasons rather than medical necessity. However, it is believed to protect against the development of **cancer** of the penis and that women with circumcised partners are at less risk from cancer of the cervix.

> ❝ When they circumcised Herbert Samuel they threw away the wrong bit. ❞
>
> **David Lloyd George**, attributed remark, *The Listener*, 7 September 1978.

CJD
Abbreviation for the fatal brain disorder Creutzfeldt–Jakob disease. One of a group of diseases characterized by spongy changes in brain tissue, CJD causes progressive physical and mental deterioration, leading to death usually within about a year of onset. Historically, CJD has been a rare disease, affecting only one in a million people. However, the UK is witnessing a slight increase with the appearance of a new variant of the disease (vCJD) which is said to be attributable to consumption of meat from **BSE**-infected cattle. There have been instances of classical CJD in people treated with pituitary **hormones** for growth or fertility problems.

cleft palate
Fissure of the roof of the mouth, often accompanied by a harelip, the result of the two halves of the palate failing to join properly during embryonic development. It can be remedied by plastic surgery. Approximately 1 child in 2,000 is born with a cleft palate. The chances of having a baby with a cleft palate are increased by smoking, taking Valium, or undergoing high stress levels.

clot-buster
Popular term for a small group of thrombolytic (clot-dissolving) drugs used in the treatment of **heart attack**. Tissue plasminogen activator (TPA) is a natural clot-buster found in the bloodstream.

cocaine

Alkaloid extracted from the leaves of the coca tree. It has limited medical application, mainly as a local **anaesthetic** agent that is readily absorbed by **mucous membranes** (lining tissues) of the nose and throat. It is both toxic and

Cocaine was first extracted from the coca plant in Germany in the 19th century. Most of the world's cocaine is produced from coca grown in Peru, Bolivia, Colombia, and Ecuador.

addictive. Its use as a stimulant is illegal. Crack is a derivative of cocaine.

Side effects of cocaine use include spasm of the conorary artery causing chest pain. Long-term use may cause mental and physical deterioration.

> ❝'For me', said Sherlock Holmes, 'there still remains the cocaine bottle'. ❞
>
> **Sir Arthur Conan Doyle**, *The Sign of Four.*

COCAINE USE

Cocaine speeds up the growth of certain insects. This enables forensic entomologists, who study insects on and around the corpse, to determine if a corpse is that of a cocaine user.

coeliac disease

Disease in which the small **intestine** fails to digest and absorb food. The disease can appear at any age but has a peak incidence in the 30–50 age group; it is more common in women. It is caused by an intolerance to gluten (a constituent of wheat, rye, and barley) and characterized by **diarrhoea** and **malnutrition**. Treatment is by a gluten-free diet.

cold, common

Minor disease of the upper respiratory tract, caused by a variety of **viruses**. Symptoms are headache, chill, nasal discharge, sore throat, and (occasionally) cough. Research indicates that the virulence of a cold depends on psychological factors and either a reduction or an increase of social or work activity, as a result of stress, in the previous six months.

> 6 Whiskey is the most popular of all remedies that won't cure the cold. 9
>
> **Jerry Vale**, *Bartlett's Unfamiliar Quotations.*

colic

Spasmodic attack of pain in the abdomen, usually coming in waves. Colicky pains are caused by the painful muscular contraction and subsequent distension of a hollow organ; for example, the bowel (intestinal colic), **gall bladder** (biliary colic), or ureter (renal colic). Infantile colic is usually due to wind in the **intestine**.

colitis

Inflammation of the colon (large intestine) with **diarrhoea** (often bloody). It is usually due to infection or some types of bacterial **dysentery**.

colostomy

Operation to bring part of the colon through the abdominal wall to the exterior in order to bypass the lower bowel. The site of the colostomy varies with the condition. The colostomy opening (stoma) is covered by an appliance to contain faecal (see **faeces**) matter. A colostomy may be temporary or permanent.

colour blindness

Hereditary defect of vision that reduces the ability to discriminate certain colours, usually red and green. The condition is sex-linked, affecting men more than women.

coma
A state of deep unconsciousness from which the subject cannot be roused. Possible causes include head injury, brain disease, liver, cerebral haemorrhage, or drug overdose.

conjunctivitis
Inflammation of the conjunctiva, the delicate membrane that lines the inside of the eyelids and covers the front of the eye. Symptoms include redness, swelling, and a watery or pus-filled discharge. Conjunctivitis may be caused by infection, **allergy**, or other irritant.

connective tissue
Tissue made up of a noncellular substance, the extracellular matrix, in which some cells are embedded. **Skin**, **bones**, **tendons**, **cartilage**, and adipose tissue (**fat**) are the main connective tissues. There are small amounts of connective tissue in organs such as the **brain** and **liver**, where they maintain the organ's shape and structure.

constipation
The infrequent emptying of the bowel. The intestinal contents are propelled by peristaltic contractions of the **intestine** in the digestive process. The faecal residue collects in the rectum, distending it and promoting defecation. Constipation may be due to illness, alterations in food consumption, stress, or as an adverse effect of certain drugs. An increased intake of dietary fibre can alleviate constipation. **Laxatives** may be used to relieve temporary constipation but they should not be used routinely.

contraceptive
Any drug, device, or technique that prevents **pregnancy**. The use of any contraceptive is part of family planning (birth control). The effectiveness of a contraceptive method is often given as a percentage. To say that a method has 95% effectiveness means that, on average, out of 100 healthy couples using that method for a year, 95 will not conceive.

TYPES OF CONTRACEPTION

- The contraceptive **Pill** contains female **hormones** that interfere with egg production or the first stage of pregnancy.
- The 'morning-after' pill can be taken up to 72 hours after unprotected intercourse.
- Barrier contraceptives include condoms (sheaths) and diaphragms, also called caps or Dutch caps; they prevent the sperm entering the cervix (neck of the womb).
- Intrauterine devices, also known as **IUDs** or coils, cause a slight inflammation of the lining of the womb; this prevents the fertilized egg from becoming implanted.
- Other contraceptive methods include **sterilization** (women) and **vasectomy** (men).
- 'Natural' methods include withdrawal of the penis before ejaculation (coitus interruptus) and avoidance of intercourse at the time of ovulation (rhythm method). These methods are unreliable and normally only used on religious grounds.

❝ It is now quite lawful for a Catholic woman to avoid pregnancy by a resort to mathematics, though she is still forbidden to resort to physics and chemistry. ❞

H L Mencken, US journalist, *Notebooks*.

convulsion
Series of violent contractions of the muscles over which the patient has no control. It may be associated with loss of consciousness. Convulsions may arise from any one of a number of causes, including brain disease (such as **epilepsy**), injury, high fever, poisoning, and electrocution.

coronary artery disease

(Latin *corona* 'crown', from the arteries encircling the heart) Condition in which the fatty deposits of **atherosclerosis** form in the coronary arteries that supply the heart muscle, narrowing them and restricting the blood flow. These arteries may already be hardened (**arteriosclerosis**). If the heart's oxygen requirements are increased, as during exercise, the blood supply through the narrowed arteries may be inadequate, and the pain of **angina** results. A **heart attack** occurs if the blood supply to an area of the heart is cut off, for example because a blood clot (thrombus) has blocked one of the coronary arteries. The subsequent lack of oxygen damages the heart muscle, and, if a large area of the heart is affected, the attack may be fatal. Coronary artery disease tends to run in families and is also linked to **smoking**, lack of exercise, and a diet high in saturated **fats** (see also **cholesterol**). A number of interventions have been tried for coronary artery disease. Most effective is bypass surgery – an operation called coronary artery bypass grafting (CABG) – to replace narrowed sections of artery.

corticosteroid

Any of several steroid **hormones** secreted by the cortex of the adrenal glands; also synthetic forms with similar properties. Corticosteroids have anti-inflammatory and immunosuppressive effects and may be used to treat a number of conditions, including **rheumatoid arthritis**, severe **allergies**, asthma, some skin diseases, and some **cancers**. Side effects can be serious and therapy must be withdrawn gradually.

The two main groups of corticosteroids are:

- glucocorticoids, which are essential to carbohydrate, fat, and protein metabolism and to the body's response to stress;
- mineralocorticoids, which regulate the balance of water and salt in the body.

cot death or sudden infant death syndrome (SIDS)

Death of an apparently healthy baby, almost always during sleep. It is most common in the winter months, and strikes more boys than girls. The cause is not known but risk factors that have been identified include prematurity, respiratory infection, overheating in the baby, and sleeping position. There was a 60% reduction in the number of cot deaths in the UK in the first nine months of 1993 following a massive advertising campaign advising parents to put their babies to sleep on their backs, ensure they do not overheat, and avoid smoking near them. However, two children in a thousand still die annually from the condition in Britain, making this the leading cause of death for children under six months of age.

cramp
Painful contraction of one or more muscles. It may be due to inadequate blood flow, fatigue, stress, or poor posture, or, more rarely, to an imbalance of mineral salts.

cranial osteopathy or craniosacral therapy
In **alternative medicine**, gentle manipulation of the cranial bones to correct displacements that may be caused by, among other things, blows to the head or dental work. It was developed in the USA in the 1920s by William Sutherland and is usually practised as a specialization by some osteopaths. Practitioners use the technique to benefit the whole nervous system and have found it effective against high **blood pressure**, headaches, and stomach ulcers.

In the 1980s a group of practitioners developed a way of using the technique to help young babies, especially those who have had 'difficult' births, '**colicky**' babies, and those with other symptoms of distress generally show a marked improvement.

Crohn's disease
(Or regional ileitis) Chronic inflammatory bowel disease. It tends to flare up for a few days at a time, causing **diarrhoea**, abdominal **cramps**, loss of appetite, weight loss, and mild **fever**. The cause of Crohn's disease is unknown, although stress may be a factor. Crohn's disease may occur in any part of the digestive system but usually affects the small **intestine**. It is characterized by ulceration, abscess formation, small perforations, and the development of adhesions

binding the loops of the small intestine. Affected segments of intestine may constrict, causing obstruction, or may perforate. It is treated by surgical removal of badly affected segments and by **corticosteroids**. Mild cases respond to rest, bland diet, and drug treatment. Crohn's disease first occurs most often in adults aged 20–40.

crystal therapy

In **alternative medicine**, application of crystals to diseased or disordered physical structures or processes to bring about healing or stabilization. Different gemstones are used as stimulators, balancers, tranquillizers, and amplifiers of healing processes, and some therapists seek to augment their effects by focusing light through the crystals or stimulating them electrically. Although healing properties have long been attributed to crystals and gemstones, the development of these therapies is recent.

cyst

Hollow cavity in the body lined with epithelium and usually filled with fluid. Cysts may be normal, for example the urinary bladder, or pathological, for example an ovarian cyst.

cystic fibrosis

Hereditary disease involving defects of various tissues, including the sweat glands, the mucous glands of the bronchi (air passages), and the **pancreas**. The sufferer experiences repeated chest infections and digestive disorders and generally fails to thrive. In 1989 a gene for cystic fibrosis was identified by teams of researchers in

Cystic fibrosis is seen as a promising test case for **gene therapy**, although early results of trials have been disappointing.

Michigan, USA, and Toronto, Canada, enabling the development of a screening test for carriers; the disease can also be detected in the unborn child.

One person in 22 is a carrier of the disease. If both parents are carriers, each of their children has a one-in-four chance of having the disease. It is the commonest fatal hereditary disease among white people, occurring in about one in 2,000 pregnancies. Cystic fibrosis was once universally fatal at an early age; now, although there is no definitive cure, treatments have raised both the quality and expectancy of life. Management of cystic fibrosis is by diet and drugs, physiotherapy to keep the chest clear, and use of **antibiotics** to combat infection and minimize damage to the lungs. Some sufferers have benefited from lung or heart-lung transplants.

cystitis

Inflammation of the **bladder**, usually caused by bacterial infection and resulting in frequent and painful urination. It is more common in women. Treatment is by **antibiotics** and drinking copious fluids containing vitamin C.

Cystitis is more common after sexual intercourse. It is thought that intercourse encourages **bacteria**, especially *Escherichia coli*, which are normally present on the skin around the anus and vagina, to enter the urethra and ascend to the bladder. By drinking water before intercourse, and passing urine afterwards, the incidence of cystitis can be reduced.

cytotoxic drug

Any drug used to kill the cells of a malignant **tumour**; it may also damage healthy cells. Side effects include nausea, vomiting, hair loss, and bone-marrow damage. Some cytotoxic drugs are also used to treat other diseases and to suppress rejection of an organ in **transplant** patients.

deafness

Partial or total deficit of hearing in either ear. Methods to overcome the disability include:

- hearing aids
- lip-reading
- a cochlear implant in the ear in combination with a special electronic processor
- sign language
- 'cued speech' (manual clarification of ambiguous lip movement during speech).

Approximately 10% of people worldwide experience some hearing difficulties. This amounts to approximately 28 million people in the USA alone.

- Conductive deafness is due to faulty conduction of sound inwards from the external ear, usually due to infection, or a hereditary abnormality of the bones of the inner ear.
- Perceptive deafness may be inborn or caused by injury or disease of the cochlea, auditory nerve, or the hearing centres in the brain. It becomes more common with age.

death

Cessation of all life functions so that the molecules and structures associated with living things become disorganized and indistinguishable from similar molecules found in nonliving things. Death used to be pronounced upon the permanent cessation of the **heartbeat** but the advent of life-support equipment has made this final stage sometimes difficult to determine. Consequently, a person may be pronounced dead when the brain ceases to control the vital functions, even if breathing and heartbeat are maintained artificially.

> ❝I am ready to meet my Maker. Whether my Maker is prepared for the ordeal of meeting me is another matter.❞
>
> **Winston Churchill**, said on his 75th birthday.

dehydration
Shortage of water in the body tissues. Symptoms include nausea, thirst, and exhaustion. It may arise from inadequate fluid intake or from excessive fluid loss (through sweating, vomiting, **diarrhoea**). It is treated by drinking plenty of fluid or by saline infusion (replacing lost salts along with water intravenously).

delirium
A state of acute confusion in which the subject is incoherent, frenzied, and out of touch with reality. It is often accompanied by delusions or hallucinations. Delirium may occur in feverish illness, some forms of mental illness, brain disease, or as a result of drug or alcohol intoxication. In chronic **alcoholism**, attacks of delirium tremens (DTs), marked by **hallucinations**, sweating, trembling, and **anxiety**, may persist for several days.

dementia
Mental deterioration as a result of physical changes in the brain. It may be due to degenerative change, circulatory disease, infection, injury, or chronic poisoning. **Senile dementia**, a progressive loss of mental faculties such as memory and orientation, is typically a disease process of old age and can be accompanied by depression.

dentistry
Care and treatment of the teeth and gums. Orthodontics deals with the straightening of the teeth (see **tooth**) for aesthetic and clinical reasons, and periodontics (see **periodontal disease**) with care of the supporting tissue (bone and gums).

The **bacteria** that start the process of dental decay are normal, nonpathogenic members of a large and varied group of micro-organisms present in the mouth. They are strains of oral strepto-

Since 1945 there has been a significant improvement in dental health in the UK. In 1988, 21% of adults had no natural teeth (30% in 1978), and, on average, each adult had 8.4 filled teeth.

cocci, and it is only in the presence of sucrose (from refined sugar) in the mouth that they become damaging to the teeth. The introduction of fluoride in the water supply has been one attempt to prevent tooth decay. However, the safety aspects of this method have come under scrutiny.

The earliest dental school was opened in Baltimore, Maryland, USA in 1839. In the UK the predecessors of the modern University College Hospital Dental School and Royal Dental Hospital and School, both within the University of London, were established in 1859 and 1860. An International Dental Federation was founded in 1900.

> ❝ It is necessary to clean the teeth frequently, more especially after meals, but not on any account with a pin, or the point of a penknife, and it must never be done at table. ❞
>
> **St Jean Baptiste de la Salle**, *The Rules of Christian Manners and Civility*.

depression

An emotional state characterized by sadness, unhappy thoughts, apathy, and dejection. Sadness is a normal response to major losses such as bereavement or unemployment. After childbirth, postnatal depression is common. Clinical depression, which is prolonged or unduly severe, often requires treatment, such as **antidepressant** medication, cognitive therapy, or, in very rare cases, **electroconvulsive therapy** (ECT), in which an electrical current is passed through the brain.

Periods of depression may alternate with periods of high optimism, over-enthusiasm, and confidence. This is the manic phase in a disorder known as manic depression or bipolar disorder. A manic depressive state is one in which a person switches repeatedly from one extreme to the other. Each mood can last for weeks or months. Typically, the depressive state lasts longer than the manic phase.

> ❝ The world leans on us. When we sag, the whole world seems to droop. ❞
>
> **Eric Hoffer**, US Philosopher, *The Passionate State of Mind.*

diabetes or diabetes mellitus

A disorder in the cells called the islets of Langerhans in the **pancreas** which prevents the body producing the hormone **insulin** so that sugars cannot be used properly; or when the body's cells fail to respond to insulin that is produced. Treatment is by dietary control and oral or injected insulin. Without treatment, the patient may lapse into diabetic **coma** and die.

There are two forms of diabetes:

- Type 1, or insulin-dependent diabetes, which usually begins in childhood and is an autoimmune condition; and the far more common form of the disease (up to 80% of all cases).

- Type 2, or noninsulin-dependent diabetes, which occurs in later life (late onset). Relatives of people with diabetes are at increased risk of developing the disease.

Careful management, including control of high **blood pressure**, can delay some of the serious complications, which include blindness, disease of the peripheral blood vessels, and kidney failure. Pancreas transplantation is sometimes undertaken for severe diabetes. Successful transplantation of insulin-producing islet cells into diabetic patients was reported in spring 2000.

Worldwide there has been a dramatic increase in the incidence of diabetes in the past three decades.

diagnosis

Determining the nature of a patient's disease or injury by consideration of signs and symptoms (elicited by examination and questioning), together with any test results, X-rays, or scans, and a knowledge of the patient's medical history.

> ❝ Declare the past, diagnose the present, foretell the future. ❞
>
> **Hippocrates**, *Epidemics.*

dialysis

Technique for removing waste products from the blood in chronic or acute **kidney** failure. There are two main methods, haemodialysis and peritoneal dialysis. In haemodialysis, the patient's blood is passed through a pump, where it is separated from sterile dialysis fluid by a semipermeable membrane. This allows any toxic substances which have built up in the bloodstream, and which would normally be filtered out by the kidneys, to diffuse out of the blood into the dialysis fluid. Haemodialysis is very expensive and usually requires the patient to attend a specialized unit.

Peritoneal dialysis uses one of the body's natural semipermeable membranes for the same purpose. About two litres of dialysis fluid is slowly instilled into the peritoneal cavity of the abdomen, and drained out again, over about two hours. During that time **toxins** from the blood diffuse into the peritoneal cavity across the peritoneal membrane. The advantage of peritoneal dialysis is that the patient can remain active while the dialysis is proceeding. This is known as continuous ambulatory peritoneal dialysis (CAPD). In the long term, dialysis is expensive and debilitating, and a **transplant** is now the treatment of choice for chronic kidney failure.

diarrhoea

Frequent or excessive action of the bowels so that the **faeces** are liquid or semiliquid. It is caused by intestinal irritants (including some drugs and poisons), infection with harmful organisms (as in **dysentery**, salmonella, or cholera), or **allergies**. Dehydration as a result of diarrhoeal disease can be treated with a solution of salt and glucose taken orally in large quantities (to restore the elec-

The World Health Organisation (WHO) reported that 3.1 million deaths had been caused by diarrhoeal disease during 1995.

trolyte balance in the blood). Since most diarrhorea is viral in origin, antibiotics are ineffective.

diet

Range of foods eaten each day; it is also a particular selection of food, or the total amount and choice of food for a specific person or people. Seven kinds of food are required for a balanced diet:

- **proteins**
- **carbohydrates**
- **fats**
- **vitamins**
- minerals
- water
- **roughage**.

Dietetics is the science of feeding individuals or groups; a dietitian is a specialist in this science. An adequate diet is one that supplies the body's daily nutritional needs (see **nutrition**) and provides sufficient energy to meet individual levels of activity. The average daily requirement for men is 2,500 calories, but this will vary with age, occupation, and weight; in general, women need fewer calories than men. The energy requirements of active children increase steadily with age, reaching a peak in the late teens. There are a number of reasons why a special diet may be adopted or advised. It may be medically recommended in order to balance, increase, or limit certain nutrients or to lose weight by a reduction in caloric intake or selection of specific foods. Special diets may also be observed on religious or moral grounds.

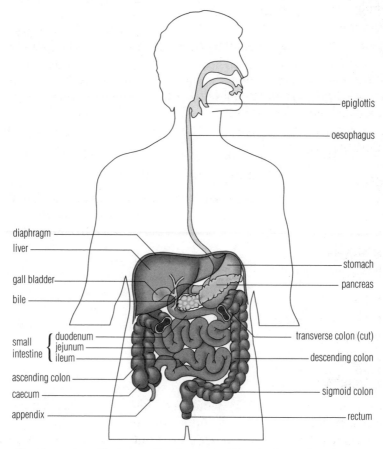

epiglottis

oesophagus

diaphragm

liver

gall bladder

bile

stomach

pancreas

small intestine { duodenum
jejunum
ileum

ascending colon

caecum

appendix

transverse colon (cut)

descending colon

sigmoid colon

rectum

digestive system *The human digestive system. When food is swallowed, it is moved down the oesophagus by the action of muscles (peristalsis) into the stomach. Digestion starts in the stomach as the food is mixed with enzymes and strong acid. After several hours, the food passes to the small intestine. Here more enzymes are added and digestion is completed. After all nutrients have been absorbed, the indigestible parts pass into the large intestine and thence to the rectum. The liver has many functions, such as storing minerals and vitamins and making bile, which is stored in the gall bladder until needed for the digestion of fats. The pancreas supplies enzymes. The appendix appears to have no function in human beings.*

digestive system

Mouth, stomach, intestine, and associated glands, all of which are involved in the digestion of food. The food is broken down by physical and chemical means in the stomach; digestion is completed and most nutrients are absorbed in the small intestine. What remains is stored and concentrated into **faeces** in the large intestine.

> 6 The fate of a nation has often depended upon the good or bad digestion of a prime minister. 9
>
> **Voltaire**, *Bartlett's Unfamiliar Quotations.*

digitalis

Drug that increases the efficiency of the heart by strengthening its muscle contractions and slowing its rate. It is derived from the leaves of the common European woodland plant *Digitalis purpurea* (foxglove).

Following the account of its properties by William Withering, an English physician and botanist, in 1785, digitalis became the first cardiac drug.

diphtheria

Acute infectious disease in which a membrane forms in the throat (threatening death by asphyxia), along with the production of a powerful toxin that damages the heart and nerves. It is treated with antitoxin and antibiotics. Although its incidence has been reduced greatly by immunization, an epidemic in the former Soviet Union resulted in 47,802 cases and 1,746 deaths in 1994, and 1,500 deaths in 1995.

- In 1995 the World Health Organization (WHO) declared the epidemic 'an international public health emergency' after 20 linked cases were identified in other parts of Europe.
- The epidemic showed signs of abating in 1996, with a 59%

decrease in the number of cases for the first three months, compared with the same period in 1995.

diuretic
Any drug that increases the output of urine by the **kidneys.** It may be used in the treatment of high **blood pressure** and to relieve oedema associated with heart, lung, kidney, or liver disease, and some **endocrine** disorders.

DNA
Abbreviation for deoxyribonucleic acid, the complex giant molecule that contains, in chemically coded form, the information needed for a **cell** to make **proteins**. DNA is a ladderlike double-stranded nucleic acid which forms the basis of genetic inheritance in all organisms, except for a few viruses that have only **RNA** (ribonucleic acid). DNA is organized into **chromosomes** and is found only in the cell nucleus. Because proteins are the chief structural molecules of living matter and, as enzymes, regulate all aspects of **metabolism**, it may be seen that the genetic code is effectively responsible for building and controlling the whole body.

Down's syndrome
Condition caused by a chromosomal abnormality (the presence of an extra copy of **chromosome** 21), which in humans produces mental retardation; a flattened face; coarse, straight hair; and a fold of skin at the inner edge of the eye (hence the former name 'mongolism'). The condition can be detected by prenatal testing (see **amniocentisis**). The incidence of Down's syndrome births in developed countries is one in 700 live births. Mothers aged over 40 are more likely to give birth to a Down's syndrome child, and in 1995 French

All people with Down's syndrome who live long enough eventually develop early-onset **Alzheimer's disease**, a form of **dementia**. This known association led to the discovery in 1991 that some forms of early-onset Alzheimer's disease are caused by a gene defect on chromosome 21.

researchers discovered a link between Down's syndrome incidence and paternal age, with men over 40 having an increased likelihood of fathering a Down's syndrome baby. The syndrome is named after J L H Down (1828–1896), an English physician who studied it.

drug and alcohol dependence

Physical or psychological craving for addictive drugs such as alcohol, nicotine, **narcotics**, tranquillizers, or stimulants. Such substances can alter mood or behaviour. When dependence is established, sudden withdrawal from the drug can cause unpleasant physical and/or psychological reactions which may be dangerous.

See also: *alcoholism.*

dysentery

Infection of the large **intestine** causing abdominal **cramps** and painful **diarrhoea** with blood. There are two kinds of dysentery:

- amoebic (caused by a protozoan), common in the tropics, which may lead to **liver** damage;
- bacterial, the kind most often seen in the temperate zones.

Both forms are successfully treated with antibacterials and fluids to prevent dehydration.

dyslexia

Malfunction in the brain's synthesis and interpretation of written information, popularly known as 'word blindness'. Dyslexia may be described as specific or developmental to distinguish it from reading or writing difficulties which are acquired. It results in poor ability in reading and writing, though the person may excel in other areas, for example, in mathematics. Acquired dyslexia may occur as a result of brain injury or disease.

In 1994 US researchers linked the occurrence of dyslexia in families to a region on chromosome 6.

ear

Organ of hearing. It responds to the vibrations that constitute sound, which are translated into nerve signals and passed to the brain. The ear consists of three parts. The outer ear is a funnel that collects sound, directing it down a tube to the ear drum (tympanic membrane), which separates the outer and middle ear. Sounds vibrate this membrane, the mechanical movement of which is transferred to a

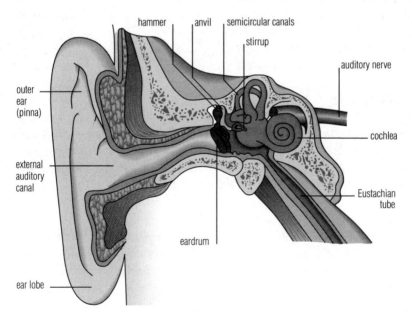

ear *The structure of the ear. The three bones of the middle ear – hammer, anvil, and stirrup – vibrate in unison and magnify sounds about 20 times. The spiral-shaped cochlea is the organ of hearing. As sound waves pass down the spiral tube, they vibrate fine hairs lining the tube, which activate the auditory nerve connected to the brain. The semicircular canals are the organs of balance, detecting movements of the head.*

smaller membrane leading to the inner ear by three small bones, the
auditory ossicles. Vibrations of the inner ear membrane move fluid
contained in the snail-shaped cochlea, which vibrates hair cells that
stimulate the auditory nerve connected to the brain. Three fluid-filled
canals of the inner ear detect changes of position; this mechanism,
with other sensory inputs, is responsible for the sense of balance.

ECG
Abbreviation for electrocardiogram, a graphic recording of the
heart's electrical activity, as detected by electrodes placed on the
skin. Electrocardiography is used in the diagnosis of **heart disease**.

ecstasy (MDMA)
An illegal drug in increasing
use from the 1980s. It is a
modified **amphetamine** with
mild psychedelic effects and
works by depleting **serotonin**
(a neurotransmitter) in the
brain. Its long-term effects are
unknown, but animal

> In the UK the annual death rate
> through ecstasy is six per year. Most of
> these deaths occur at clubs or raves
> where dehydration and over heating is
> a major factor.

experiments have shown brain damage. Ecstasy was first synthesized
in 1914 by the Merck pharmaceutical company in Germany. It was
one of eight psychedelics tested by the US army in 1953 but was
otherwise largely forgotten until the mid-1970s.

eczema
Inflammatory skin condition, a form of dermatitis, marked by dry-
ness, rashes, itching, the formation of blisters, and the exudation of
fluid. It may be allergic (see **allergy**) in origin and is sometimes complicated by infection. Treatment depends on the cause but usually
involves use of a **corticosteroid** ointment.

EEG
Abbreviation for electroencephalogram, a graphic record of the
electrical discharges of the brain as detected by electrodes placed

on the scalp. The pattern of electrical activity revealed by electroencephalography is helpful in the diagnosis of some brain disorders, in particular **epilepsy**.

Ehrlich, Paul (1854–1915)
German bacteriologist and immunologist who discovered salvarsan, the first cure for **syphilis**. He combed through the arsenic compounds to find salvarsan, used in the treatment of the disease before the discovery of **antibiotics**. He shared the 1908 Nobel Prize for Physiology or Medicine with the Russian microbiologist Ilya Metchnikoff (1845–1916) for work on **immunization**.

electroconvulsive therapy or ECT or electroshock therapy
Treatment administered mainly for severe depression, given under anaesthesia and with a muscle relaxant. An electric current is passed through one or both sides of the brain to induce alterations in its electrical activity. The treatment can cause distress and loss of concentration and memory, and so there is much controversy about its use and effectiveness.

ECT was first used in 1938 but its success in treating depression led to its excessive use for a wide range of mental illnesses against which it was ineffective. Its side effects included broken bones and severe memory loss. The procedure in use today is much improved, using the minimum shock necessary to produce a seizure, administered under general anaesthetic with muscle relaxants to prevent muscle spasms and fractures.

embolism
Blockage of a blood vessel by an obstruction called an embolus (usually a blood clot, fat particle, or bubble of air).

embryo
Early developmental stage following **fertilization** of an ovum (egg cell) produced by an **ovary**. The term embryo describes the fertilized egg during its first seven weeks of existence; from the eighth week onwards it is referred to as a **fetus**.

embryo *The development of a bird and a human embryo. In the human, division of the fertilized egg, or ovum, begins within hours of conception. Within a week, a hollow, fluid-containing ball – a blastocyte – with a mass of cells at one end has developed. After the third week, the embryo has changed from a mass of cells into a recognizable shape. At four weeks, the embryo is 3 mm/0.1 in long, with a large bulge for the heart and small pits for the ears. At six weeks, the embryo is 1.5 cm/0.6 in long with a pulsating heart and ear flaps. By the eighth week, the embryo (now technically a fetus) is 2.5 cm/1 in long and recognizably human, with eyelids and small fingers and toes.*

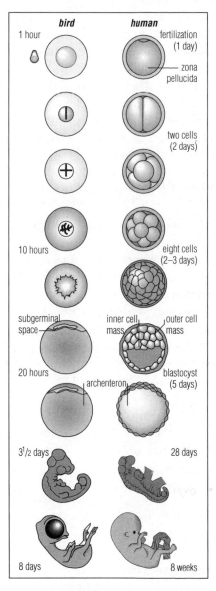

embryology

Study of the growth and development of the **embryo** and **fetus** from the time of **fertilization** until birth. It is mainly concerned with the changes in cell organization in the embryo and the way in which these lead to the structures and organs of the adult.

emphysema

Incurable lung condition characterized by disabling breathlessness. Progressive loss of the thin walls dividing the air spaces (alveoli) in the **lungs** reduces the area available for the exchange of oxygen and carbon dioxide, causing the lung tissue to expand. The term 'emphysema' can also refer to the presence of air in other body tissues. Emphysema is most often seen at an advanced stage of chronic **bronchitis**, although it may develop in other long-standing diseases of the lungs. It destroys lung tissue, leaving behind air blisters called bullae. As the disease progresses, the bullae occupy more and more space in the chest cavity, inflating the lungs and causing severe breathing difficulties. The bullae may be removed surgically, and since early 1994 US trials have achieved measured success using lasers to eliminate them in a procedure called lung-reduction pneumoplasty (LRP).

encephalitis
Inflammation of the brain, nearly always due to viral infection but it may also occur in bacterial and other infections. It varies widely in severity, from shortlived, relatively slight effects of headache, drowsiness, and fever to paralysis, **coma**, and death.

endocrine gland
Gland that secretes **hormones** into the bloodstream to regulate body processes. The main endocrine glands are:

- the **pituitary**
- **thyroid**
- parathyroids
- adrenals
- **pancreas**
- **ovaries**
- **testes**.

See also: *exocrine gland.*

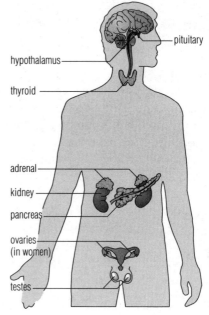

endocrine gland *The main human endocrine glands. These glands produce hormones, chemical messengers, which travel in the bloodstream to stimulate certain cells.*

endometriosis
Common gynaecological complaint in which patches of endometrium (the lining of the

womb) are found outside the **uterus**. This ectopic (abnormally positioned) tissue is present most often in the **ovaries**, although it may invade any pelvic or abdominal site, as well as the **vagina** and rectum. Endometriosis may be treated with **analgesics**, hormone preparations or surgery. Between 30% and 40% of women treated for infertility suffer from the condition.

endorphin

Natural substance (a polypeptide) that modifies the action of nerve cells. Endorphins are produced by the **pituitary gland** and hypothalamus of vertebrates. They lower the perception of pain by reducing the transmission of signals between nerve cells. Endorphins regulate pain, hunger, and are involved in the release of sex hormones from the pituitary gland. Opiates act in a similar way to endorphins, but are not rapidly degraded by the body, as natural endorphins are, and thus have a long-lasting effect on pain perception and mood. Endorphin release is stimulated by exercise.

endoscopy

Examination of internal organs or tissues by an instrument allowing direct vision. An endoscope is equipped with an eyepiece, lenses, and its own light source to illuminate the field of vision. The endoscope used to examine the digestive tract is a flexible fibreoptic instrument swallowed by the patient. There are various types of endoscope in use – some rigid, some flexible – with names prefixed by their site of application (for example, bronchoscope and laryngoscope). The value of endoscopy is in permitting diagnosis without the need for exploratory surgery. **Biopsies** (tissue samples) and photographs may be taken by way of the endoscope as an aid to diagnosis, or to monitor the effects of treatment. Some surgical procedures can be performed using fine instruments introduced through the endoscope (see **keyhole surgery**).

epilepsy

Medical disorder characterized by a tendency to develop fits, which are **convulsions** or abnormal feelings caused by abnormal electrical discharges in the cerebral hemispheres of the brain. Epilepsy can be controlled with a number of anticonvulsant drugs.

The term epilepsy covers a range of conditions from mild 'absences', involving momentary loss of awareness, to major convulsions. In some cases the abnormal electrical activity is focal (confined to one area of the brain); in others it is generalized throughout the **cerebral cortex**. Fits are classified according to their clinical type. They include:

- the *grand mal* seizure with convulsions and loss of consciousness;
- the fleeting absence of awarenes *petit mal*, almost exclusively a disorder of childhood;
- Jacksonian seizures, originating in the motor cortex;
- and temporal-lobe fits, which may be associated with visual hallucinations and bizarre disturbances of the sense of smell.

Epilepsy affects between 1% and 3% of the world's population. It may arise spontaneously or may be a consequence of brain surgery, organic brain disease, head injury, metabolic disease, **alcoholism**, or withdrawal from some drugs. Almost a third of patients have a family history of the condition.

Escherichia coli (E. coli)

Rod-shaped Gram-negative bacterium (see **bacteria**) that lives, usually harmlessly, in the colon of most warm-blooded animals. It is the commonest cause of urinary tract infections in humans. It is sometimes found in water or meat where faecal contamination has occurred and can cause severe gastric problems.

The mapping of the genome of E. coli, consisting of 4,403 genes, was completed in 1997. It is probably the organism about which most molecular genetics is known, and is of preeminent importance in recombinant DNA research.

euthanasia

Mercy killing of someone with a severe and incurable condition or illness. Euthanasia is an issue that creates much controversy on medical and ethical grounds. A patient's right to refuse life-prolonging treatment is recognized in several countries.

- In Australia, a bill legalizing voluntary euthanasia for terminally ill patients was passed by the Northern Territory state legislature in May 1995. This law was overturned in March 1997; four people had died, all having suffered from terminal cancer.
- In the Netherlands, where approximately 2,700 patients formally request it each year, euthanasia is technically illegal. However, provided guidelines issued by the Royal Dutch Medical Association are strictly adhered to, doctors are not prosecuted.

> 6 Death is not the greatest of ills, it is worse to want to die, and not to be able to. 9
>
> **Sophocles**, *Electra*.

evening primrose oil

Oil from any plant of the genus *Oenothera*, family Onagraceae. It is rich in gamma-linoleic acid (GLA). The body converts GLA into substances which resemble **hormones**, and evening primrose oil is beneficial in relieving the symptoms of **premenstrual tension**. It is also used in treating **eczema** and chronic fatigue syndrome.

exocrine gland

Gland that discharges secretions, usually through a tube or a duct, on to a surface. Examples include sweat glands which release sweat on to the skin and digestive glands which release digestive juices on to the walls of the intestine.

See also: *endocrine glands.*

eye

The organ of vision. In the eye, the light is focused by the combined action of the curved cornea, the internal fluids, and the lens. Light enters the eye through the cornea and passes through the circular

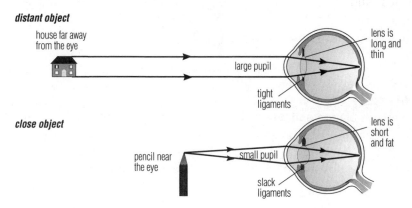

distant object

house far away
from the eye

lens is
long and
thin

large pupil

tight
ligaments

close object

lens is
short
and fat

pencil near
the eye

small pupil

slack
ligaments

eye *The mechanism by which the shape of the lens in the eye is changed so that clear images of objects, whether distant or near, can be focused on the retina.*

opening (pupil) in the iris (the coloured part of the eye). The ciliary muscles act on the lens (the rounded transparent structure behind the iris) to change its shape so that images of objects at different distances can be focused on the retina. This is at the back of the eye and is packed with light-sensitive cells (rods and cones), connected to the brain by the optic nerve.

See also: *blind spot.*

faeces

Remains of food and other waste material eliminated from the digestive tract by way of the anus. Faeces consist of quantities of fibrous material, **bacteria,** and other **micro-organisms**, dislodged lining cells of the digestive tract, bile fluids, undigested food, minerals, and water.

fainting

Sudden, temporary loss of consciousness caused by reduced blood supply to the brain. It may be due to emotional shock or physical factors, such as pooling of blood in the legs from standing still for long periods.

Fallopian tube or oviduct

In females, one of the two tubes that carry eggs (ova) from the **ovary** to the **uterus**. An egg is fertilized by sperm in the Fallopian tubes, which are lined with cells whose cilia move the egg towards the uterus.

See also: *menstrual cycle, fertilization.*

fat

In the broadest sense, a mixture of lipids – chiefly triglycerides (lipids containing three fatty acid molecules linked to a molecule of glycerol). More specifically, the term refers to a lipid mixture that is solid at room temperature (20°C); lipid mixtures that are liquid at room temperature are called oils. The higher the proportion of saturated fatty acids in a mixture, the harder the fat.

Fats are essential constituents of food, with a calorific value twice that of **carbohydrates**. However, eating too much fat, especially fat of animal origin, has been linked with **heart disease**. Excess carbohydrates and **proteins** are converted into fats for storage in special-ized connective tissues (adipose tissues), which not only act as energy reserves but also insulate the body and cushion its organs. As a nutrient, fat serves five purposes:

- it is a source of energy;
- makes the diet palatable;
- provides basic building blocks for cell structure; provides essen-tial fatty acids; and
- acts as a carrier for fat-soluble **vitamins** (A, D, E, and K).

Foods rich in fat are butter, lard, margarine, and cooking oils. Products high in monounsaturated or polyunsaturated fats are thought to be less likely to contribute to cardiovascular disease.

fatty acid or carboxylic acid
Organic compound consisting of a hydrocarbon chain of an even number of carbon atoms, with a carboxyl group (-COOH) at one end. The covalent bonds between the carbon atoms may be single or double; where a double bond occurs the carbon atoms con-cerned carry one instead of two hydrogen atoms. Chains with only single bonds have all the hydrogen they can carry, so they are said to be saturated with hydrogen. Chains with one or more double bonds are said to be unsaturated. Fatty acids are produced in the small intestine when fat is digested.

femur
The thigh-bone, the longest **bone** in the body. It has a rounded head which articulates with the hip bone. The bone has two large condyles (knuckles) on its lower end which have extensive surfaces that articulate with the tibia in the knee joint. It has been shown that the adult femur can support a compressive load of about 900 kg/1,990 lb, far more than the weight of the body.

fertility drug
Any of a range of drugs taken to increase a female's fertility, devel-oped in Sweden in the mid-1950s. They increase the chances of a

multiple birth. The most familiar is gonadotrophin, which is made from **hormone** extracts taken from the human pituitary gland. It stimulates ovulation in women. As a result of a fertility drug, in 1974 the first sextuplets to survive were born to Susan Rosenkowitz of South Africa.

fertilization
Fusion of a sperm and ovum (gametes) to produce a zygote, which combines the genetic material contributed by each parent. It usually takes place in the **Fallopian tube**.

fetus
Stage in **embryo** development. The embryo is usually termed a fetus after the eighth week of development, when the limbs and external features of the head are recognizable.

fever
Condition of raised **body temperature**, usually due to infection.

first aid
Action taken immediately in a medical emergency in order to save a sick or injured person's life, prevent further damage, or facilitate later treatment. **See also:** *resuscitation*.

Fleming, Alexander (1881–1955)
Scottish bacteriologist who discovered the first antibiotic drug, **penicillin**, in 1928. He found an unusual mould growing on a culture dish, which he isolated and grew into a pure culture; this led to his discovery of penicillin. It came into use in 1941. Fleming was born in Ayrshire and studied medicine at St Mary's Hospital, London, where he remained in the bacteriology department for his entire career, becoming professor in 1928. Fleming discovered the antibacterial properties of penicillin but its purification and concentration were left to Howard W Florey and Ernst B Chain, with whom he shared the Nobel Prize for Physiology or Medicine in 1945. He identified organisms that cause wound infections and showed how cross-infection by

streptococci can occur among patients in hospital wards. He also studied the effects of different antiseptics on various kinds of **bacteria** and on living cells. His interest in **chemotherapy** led him to introduce Paul **Ehrlich's** salvarsan into UK medical practice. He was knighted in 1944.

food poisoning

Any acute illness characterized by vomiting and **diarrhoea** and caused by eating food contaminated with harmful **bacteria** (for example, listeriosis), poisonous foods (for example, certain mushrooms, puffer fish), or

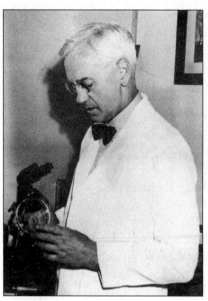

Fleming *Alexander Fleming discovered the first antibiotic drug, penicillin.*

poisoned food (such as lead or arsenic introduced accidentally during processing). A frequent cause of food poisoning is the *Salmonella* bacterium. of which strains are found in cattle, pigs, poultry, and eggs. Deep freezing of poultry before the birds are properly cooked is a common cause of food poisoning. Attacks of **salmonella** also come from contaminated eggs that have been eaten raw or cooked only lightly. Pork may carry the roundworm *Trichinella*. The most dangerous food poison is the bacillus that

---

KEBABS

In 1998 kebabs were temporarily banned in Almaty, Kazakhstan, following several cases of transmission of the disease anthrax from eating infected meat.

causes botulism. This is rare but leads to muscle paralysis and, often, death. Food irradiation is intended to prevent food poisoning.

frostbite
The freezing of skin or flesh, with formation of ice crystals leading to tissue damage. The treatment is slow warming of the affected area; for example, by skin-to-skin contact or with lukewarm water. Frostbitten parts are extremely vulnerable to infection, with the risk of **gangrene**.

frozen shoulder
Acute pain and reduced mobility in the shoulder joint. It is a common condition that may follow injury, overuse, stroke, or heart attack, or may develop for no apparent reason. It is notoriously intractable but **analgesics**, exercise or manipulation, and sometimes a **corticosteroid** injection are among treatments used to ease pain and restore mobility.

Galen (*c*.129–*c*.200)

Greek physician and anatomist whose ideas dominated Western medicine for almost 1,500 years. Galen postulated a circulation system in which the liver produced the natural spirit, the heart the vital spirit, and the brain the animal spirit. He also wrote about philosophy and believed that nature expressed a divine purpose. Galen was born in Pergamum in Asia Minor and studied medicine there and at Smyrna (now Izmir), Corinth in Greece, and Alexandria in

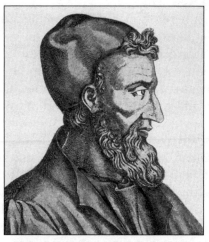

Galen *Galen's ideas dominated Western medicine for almost 1,500 years. He made important inferences about human anatomy from dissecting animals.*

Egypt, after which he returned home to become chief physician to the gladiators at Pergamum. In 161 he went to Rome, where he became a society physician and attended the Roman emperor Marcus Aurelius Antoninus. Although Galen made relatively few discoveries and relied heavily on the teachings of **Hippocrates**, he wrote a large number of books, more than 100 of which are known.

> ❝ The physician is Nature's assistant. ❞
>
> **Galen,** *Commentary on Hippocrates'* De Humoribus.

gall bladder
Small muscular sac, part of the **digestive system**. It is situated on the underside of the **liver** and connected to the small intestine by the bile duct. It stores bile from the liver.

gallstone
Pebble-like, insoluble accretion formed in the human **gall bladder** or bile ducts from cholesterol or calcium salts present in bile. Gallstones may be symptomless or they may cause pain, indigestion, or jaundice. They can be dissolved with medication or removed, either by means of an endoscope or, along with the gall bladder, in an operation known as cholecystectomy.

gangrene
Death and decay of body tissue (often a limb) due to bacterial action; the affected part turns black and causes **blood poisoning**. Gangrene sets in as a result of loss of blood supply to the area. This may be due to disease (**diabetes**, **atherosclerosis**), an obstruction of a major blood vessel (as in **thrombosis**), injury, or frostbite. Bacteria colonize the site unopposed, and a strong risk of blood poisoning often leads to surgical removal of the tissue or the affected part (amputation). Gas gangrene is caused by infection of serious wounds with the bacterium *Clostridium perfringens*. The bacterium produces a protein, alpha toxin, that destroys healthy tissue surrounding the wound. The spread is very rapid. A **vaccine** against gas gangrene was successfully tested on animals 1994.

gastroenteritis
Inflammation of the stomach and intestines, giving rise to abdominal pain, vomiting and **diarrhoea**. It may be caused by food or other poisoning, allergy, or infection. Dehydration may be severe and it is a particular risk in infants.

gene
Unit of inherited material, encoded by a strand of **DNA** and transcribed by **RNA**. Genes are located on the **chromosomes**. A gene

consistently affects a particular character in an individual – for example, the gene for eye colour. Also termed a Mendelian gene, after Austrian biologist Gregor **Mendel**, it occurs at a particular point, or locus, on a particular chromosome and may have several variants. Genes produce their visible effects simply by coding for proteins; they control the structure of those proteins via the genetic code, as well as the amounts produced and the timing of production. Genes undergo mutation and recombination to produce the variation on which natural selection operates.

gene therapy
Mode of treatment to cure or alleviate inherited diseases or defects, certain infections, and several kinds of **cancer**. The term covers a number of treatments, all involving the introduction of an artificially manipulated gene into the body to overcome a disease. The first patient to undergo gene therapy, in 1990, was a small child with severe combined immune deficiency (SCID), a rare immune disorder. At this time there were high hopes of achieving a cure for many diseases. Various methods of delivering the altered genes have been tried since, including 'packaging' them in disabled viruses. However, after many hundreds of experiments only one actual cure has been reported (also in a child with SCID). Meanwhile, this whole field remains under a cloud following the death in September 1999 of a young man receiving gene therapy for a rare metabolic disorder. This incident, and the revelations of other trials-related deaths which followed it, brought about the cancellation of some programmes and, in the USA, a tightening of controls on gene therapy experimentation.

genitalia
Reproductive organs, particularly the external/visible organs: in males, the **penis** and the scrotum, which contains the testes; in females, the clitoris and vulva.

German measles or rubella
Mild, communicable **viral** disease, usually caught by children. It is marked by a sore throat, pinkish rash, and slight fever, and has an

incubation period of two to three weeks. If a woman contracts it in the first three months of pregnancy, it may cause serious damage to the unborn child. Immunization is recommended for girls who have not contracted the disease, at about 12–14 months or at puberty.

Gerson therapy
In **alternative medicine**, radical nutritional therapy for degenerative diseases, particularly cancer, developed by German-born US physician Max Gerson (1881–1959).

ginseng
Plant with a thick, forked aromatic root used in **alternative medicine** as a tonic.

glandular fever or infectious mononucleosis
Viral disease characterized at onset by fever and painfully swollen **lymph** nodes; there may also be digestive upset, sore throat, and skin rashes. Lassitude in the patient persists for months, for years in some cases, and recovery can be slow. It is caused by the Epstein–Barr virus.

glaucoma
Condition in which pressure inside the eye (intra-ocular pressure) is raised abnormally as excess fluid accumulates. It occurs when the normal outflow of fluid within the chamber of the eye (aqueous humour) is interrupted. As pressure rises, the optic nerve suffers irreversible damage, leading to a reduction in the field of vision and, ultimately, loss of eyesight. The most common type, chronic glaucoma, usually affects people over the age of 40. It can usually be controlled by drug therapy. Laser treatment often improves drainage for a time; surgery to create an artificial channel for fluid to leave the eye offers more long-term relief. Acute glaucoma is a precipitous rise in pressure which has to be treated surgically to remove the cause of the obstruction. Acute glaucoma is extremely painful and is a medical emergency since damage to the optic nerve begins within hours of onset.

glomerulonephritis
Group of **kidney** disorders characterized by damage to the glomeruli, clusters of capillaries through which waste products are filtered out of the blood and into the kidney tubules. It is the commonest cause of end-stage kidney failure.

glue ear or secretory otitis media
Condition commonly affecting small children, in which the Eustachian tube, which normally drains and ventilates the middle **ear**, becomes blocked with **mucus**. The resulting accumulation of mucus in the middle ear muffles hearing. It is the leading cause of deafness (usually transient) in children. Glue ear resolves spontaneously after some months, but because the loss of hearing can interfere with a child's schooling the condition is often treated by a drainage procedure (myringotomy) and the surgical insertion of a small ventilating tube, or grommet, into the eardrum (tympanic membrane). The grommet is gradually extruded from the eardrum over several months and the eardrum then heals naturally.

gonorrhoea
Common **sexually transmitted disease** or **venereal disease** arising from infection with the bacterium *Neisseria gonorrhoeae*, which causes inflammation of the genito-urinary tract. After an incubation period of two to ten days, infected men experience pain while urinating and a discharge from the penis; infected women often have no external symptoms. Untreated gonorrhea carries the threat of sterility to both sexes; there is also the risk of blindness in a baby born to an infected mother. The condition is treated with **antibiotics,** though ever-increasing doses are becoming necessary to combat resistant strains of the disease.

gout
Hereditary form of arthritis, marked by an excess of uric acid crystals in the tissues, causing pain and **inflammation** in one or more joints (usually of the feet, most commonly in the big toe, or hands). Acute attacks are treated with anti-inflammatories. The disease, ten times more common in men, poses a long-term threat to the blood vessels

WHY PIGS DON'T GET GOUT

Pigs never suffer from gout. In humans the disease is caused by a build up of uric acid. Pigs have an enzyme that breaks uric acid into soluble components. Humans do not have this enzyme, so they suffer from gout and pigs do not.

and the kidneys, so ongoing treatment may be needed to minimize the levels of uric acid in the bloodstream. It is aggravated by heavy drinking.

> ❦ Oh! When I have the gout, I feel as if I was walking on my eyeballs. ❦
>
> **Sydney Smith**, *A Memoir of the Rev. Sydney Smith,* Chapter 11.

haematoma

Accumulation of blood in the tissues, causing a solid swelling. It may be due to injury, disease, or a blood clotting disorder such as **haemophilia**.

haemoglobin

Protein used for oxygen transport because the two substances combine reversibly. It occurs in **red blood cells** (erythrocytes), giving them their colour. In the lungs where the concentration of oxygen is high, oxygen attaches to haemoglobin to form oxyhaemoglobin. This process effectively increases the amount of oxygen that can be carried in the bloodstream. The oxygen is later released in the body tissues where it is at a low concentration, and the deoxygenated blood returned to the lungs.

haemophilia

Any of several inherited diseases in which normal **blood clotting** is impaired. The sufferer experiences prolonged bleeding from the slightest wound, as well as painful internal bleeding without apparent cause. Haemophilias are nearly always sex-linked, transmitted through the female line only to male infants; they have afflicted a number of European royal households. Males affected by the most common form are unable to synthesize Factor VIII, a protein involved in the clotting of blood. Treatment is primarily with Factor VIII (now mass-produced by recombinant techniques), but the haemophiliac remains at risk from the slightest incident of bleeding. The disease is a painful one that causes deformities of joints.

haemorrhoids

Distended blood vessels (**varicose veins**), in the area of the anus, popularly called **piles**.

haemorrhage
Loss of **blood** from the circulatory system. It is 'manifest' when the blood can be seen, as when it flows from a wound, and 'occult' when the bleeding is internal, as from an ulcer or internal injury.

Rapid, profuse haemorrhage causes **shock** and may prove fatal if the circulating volume cannot be replaced in time. Slow, sustained bleeding may lead to **anaemia**. Arterial bleeding is potentially more serious than blood lost from a vein. It may be stemmed by applying pressure directly to the wound.

hallucination
Perception of something that does not exist. It may be visual but may also arise from any of the other senses. Unlike an illusion, a hallucination has no basis in reality. It may occur in **psychosis**, in organic brain disease (especially temporal lobe **epilepsy**), or can be induced by some drugs.

hallucinogen
Any substance that acts on the **central nervous system** to produce changes in perception and mood and often hallucinations. Hallucinogens include LSD, peyote, and mescaline. Their effects are unpredictable and they are illegal in most countries. In some circumstances hallucinogens may produce panic or even suicidal feelings, which can recur without warning several days or months after taking the drug. In rare cases they produce an irreversible psychotic state mimicking **schizophrenia**. Spiritual or religious experiences are common, hence the ritual use of hallucinogens in some cultures. They work by chemical interference with the normal action of neurotransmitters in the brain.

Harvey, William (1578–1657)
English physician who discovered the circulation of the blood. In 1628 he published his book *De motu cordis/On the Motion of the Heart and the Blood in Animals.* Harvey's discovery mar-ked the beginning of the decline of medicine as taught by **Galen**, which had been accepted for 1,400 years.

Harvey was born in Folkestone, Kent, and studied at Cambridge and at Padua, Italy, under Geronimo Fabricius. He worked at St Bartholomew's Hospital, London, and was professor there during 1615–43. From 1618 he was court physician to James I and later to Charles I. Examining the heart and blood vessels of mammals, Harvey deduced that the

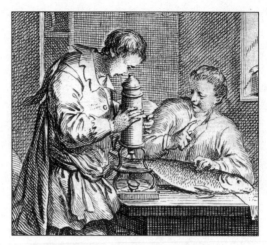

Harvey *William Harvey, English physician who discovered the circulation of blood.*

blood in the veins must flow only towards the heart. He also calculated the amount of blood that left the heart at each beat, and realized that the same blood must be circulating continuously around the body. He reasoned that it passes from the right side of the heart to the left through the lungs (pulmonary circulation).

hay fever

Allergic reaction to pollen (see **allergy**), causing sneezing, with **inflammation** of the nasal membranes, and conjunctiva of the eyes. Symptoms are due to the release of histamine. Treatment is by **antihistamine** drugs. An estimated 25% of Britons, 33% of Americans, and 40% of Australians suffer from hayfever.

Scientists prefer to call the condition seasonal rhinitis since hay fever is not caused only by grass pollen but by that of flowers and trees as well; some people also react to airborne spores and moulds which are prevalent in autumn.

> ❬ Hay Fever is the real Flower Power. ❭
>
> **Leonard Louis Levinson**, *Bartlett's Unfamiliar Quotations.*

health screening

The systematic testing for evidence of a disease, or of conditions that may precede it, in people who are at risk but not suffering from any symptoms. The aim of screening is to try to limit ill health from preventable diseases that might otherwise go undetected in the early stages. Examples are **hypothyroidism** and **phenylketonuria**, for which all newborn babies in Western countries are screened; breast cancer (screening is carried out by **mammography**), and cervical **cancer** (results of a cervical smear are analysed); and stroke, for which high **blood pressure** is a known risk factor. The criteria for a successful screening programme are:

- that the disease should be important and treatable;
- the population at risk is identifiable;
- the screening test is acceptable, accurate, and cheap;
- and that the results of screening should justify the costs involved.

heart

Muscular organ that rhythmically contracts to force **blood** around the body. It is more or less conical in shape and is positioned within the chest, behind the breast bone, above the diaphragm, and between the two lungs. A healthy heart is the size of a person's closed fist. It has four chambers – the thin-walled atria that expand to receive blood and the thick-walled ventricles that pump it out. The beating of the heart is controlled by the autonomic **nervous system** and an internal control centre or pacemaker, the sinoatrial node. The cardiac cycle is the sequence of events during

Deposits of calcium in diseased heart valves are sometimes actually bone tissue, possibly caused when heart cells follow a new developmental pathway as a result of inflammation.

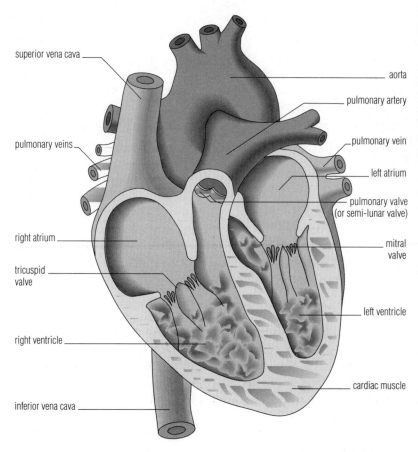

superior vena cava

aorta

pulmonary artery

pulmonary vein

pulmonary veins

left atrium

pulmonary valve
(or semi-lunar valve)

right atrium

mitral
valve

tricuspid
valve

right ventricle

left ventricle

inferior vena cava

cardiac muscle

heart *The structure of the human heart. During an average lifetime, the human heart beats more than 2,000 million times and pumps 500 million l/110 million gal of blood.*

one complete cycle of a **heartbeat**. This consists of the simultaneous contraction of the two atria, a short pause, then the simultaneous contraction of the two ventricles, followed by a longer pause while the entire heart relaxes. The contraction phase is called 'systole' and the relaxation phase which follows is called 'diastole'. The whole cycle is repeated 70–80 times a minute under resting conditions. The heart valves prevent back flow of blood.

heart attack or myocardial infarction

Sudden onset of gripping central chest pain, often accompanied by sweating and vomiting, caused by death of a portion of the heart muscle following obstruction of a coronary artery by **thrombosis** (formation of a blood clot). Half of all heart attacks result in death within the first two hours but survival in the remainder has improved following the widespread use of thrombolytic (**clot-buster**) drugs.

heartbeat

The regular contraction and relaxation of the heart and the accompanying sounds. As blood passes through the heart a double beat is heard. The first is produced by the sudden closure of the valves between the atria and the ventricles. The second, slightly delayed sound is caused by the closure of the valves found at the entrance to the major arteries leaving the heart. Diseased valves may make unusual sounds, known as heart murmurs.

heartburn

Burning sensation behind the breastbone (sternum). It results from irritation of the lower **oesophagus** (gullet) by excessively acid stomach contents, as sometimes happens during pregnancy and in cases of duodenal ulcer or **obesity**. It is often due to a weak valve at the entrance to the stomach that allows its contents to well up into the oesophagus.

heart failure

Condition arising when the heart's pumping mechanism is inadequate. It results in back pressure of blood, causing congestion of the **liver** and **lungs**, failure of the peripheral blood supply, and **oedema**. It is a consequence of damage to the heart muscle and may ensue from heart disease, especially coronary heart disease, and various other conditions, including **hypertension**, viral infection, and **thyroid** overactivity. Treatment is with **diuretics** and heart drugs.

heatstroke or sunstroke

Rise in body temperature caused by excessive exposure to heat. Mild heatstroke is experienced as feverish lassitude, sometimes with simple fainting; recovery is prompt following rest and replenishment of salt lost in sweat. Severe heatstroke causes collapse akin to that

Death rates increase by half during heatwaves; heat stress is responsible for more deaths than any meteorological cause, including cyclones and floods.

seen in acute shock and is potentially lethal without prompt treatment, including cooling the body carefully and giving fluids to relieve dehydration.

hepatitis

Any inflammatory disease of the **liver**, usually caused by a **virus**. Other causes include alcohol, drugs, gallstones, **lupus** erythematosus, and amoebic **dysentery**. Symptoms include weakness, nausea, and jaundice. Five different hepatitis viruses have been identified: A, B, C, D, and E.

- The hepatitis A virus (HAV) is the commonest cause of viral hepatitis, responsible for up to 40% of cases worldwide. It is spread by contaminated food.

  In 1998, the World Health Organization (WHO) estimated that some 350 million people were infected with hepatitis B.

- Hepatitis B, or serum hepatitis, is a highly contagious disease spread by blood products or in body fluids. It often culminates in liver failure and is also associated with liver cancer, although only 5% of those infected suffer chronic liver damage. Vaccines are available against hepatitis A and B.

- Hepatitis C is mostly seen in people needing frequent transfusions. In 1999 there were an estimated 150 million people worldwide infected with hepatitis C and 75% of these will go on to develop chronic liver infections.

- Hepatitis D, which only occurs in association with hepatitis B, is common in the Mediterranean region.

- Hepatitis E is endemic in India and South America.

herbalism

In **alternative medicine**, the prescription and use of plants and their derivatives for medication. Herbal products are favoured by alternative practitioners as 'natural medicine', as opposed to modern synthesized medicines and drugs, which are regarded with suspicion because of the dangers of side effects and dependence. Many herbal remedies are of proven efficacy both in preventing and curing illness.

heredity

The transmission of traits from parents to offspring.

> 6 The law of heredity is that all the undesirable traits come from the other parent. 9
>
> **Anon.**

hernia or rupture

Protrusion of part of an internal organ through a weakness in the surrounding muscular wall, usually in the groin. The appearance is that of a rounded soft lump or swelling.

heroin or diamorphine

Powerful opiate **analgesic**, an acetyl derivative of **morphine**. It is more addictive than morphine but causes less nausea. It has an important place in the control of severe pain in terminal illness, severe injuries, and heart attacks. It is widely used illegally. Heroin was discovered in Germany in 1898.

The major regions of opium production, for conversion to heroin, are the 'Golden Crescent' of Afghanistan, Iran, and Pakistan, and the 'Golden Triangle' across parts of Myanmar (Burma), Laos, and Thailand.

herpes

Any of several infectious diseases caused by viruses of the herpes group. Herpes simplex I is the causative agent of a common inflammation, the cold sore. Herpes simplex II is responsible for genital herpes, a highly contagious, **sexually transmitted disease** characterized by painful blisters in the **genital** area. It can be transmitted in the birth canal from mother to newborn. Herpes zoster causes **shingles**; another herpes virus causes **chickenpox**. A number of antivirals treat these infections, which are particularly troublesome in patients whose immune systems have been suppressed medically; for example, after a **transplant** operation. The drug *acyclovir*, originally introduced for the treatment of genital herpes, has now been shown to modify the course of chickenpox and the related condition shingles, by reducing the duration of the illness.

hiccup

Sharp noise caused by a sudden spasm of the diaphragm with closing of the windpipe, commonly caused by digestive disorder. On rare occasions, hiccups may become continuous, when they are very debilitating. Treatment with a muscle relaxant drug may be effective.

Hippocrates (*c.* 460– *c.* 377 BC)

Greek physician, often called the founder of medicine. Important Hippocratic ideas include cleanliness (for patients and physicians), moderation in eating and drinking, letting nature take its course, and living where the air is good. He believed that health was the result of the 'humours' of the body being in balance; imbalance caused disease. These ideas were later adopted by **Galen**.

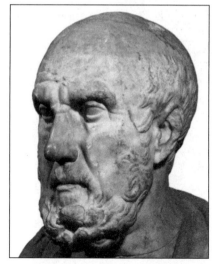

Hippocrates *Greek physician considered the founder of medical science.*

Hippocrates was born on the island of Kos, where he also practised and founded a medical school. He travelled throughout Greece and Asia Minor and died in Thessaly.

The *Corpus Hippocraticum/ Hippocratic Collection*, a group of some 70 works, is attributed to him but was probably not written by him, although the works outline his approach to medicine. They include *Aphorisms* and the *Hippocratic Oath*, which embodies the essence of medical ethics.

❝ We must turn to nature itself, to the observations of the body in health and disease to learn the truth. ❞

Hippocrates, *Aphorisms*.

Hodgkin's disease or lymphadenoma

Rare form of **cancer** mainly affecting the **lymph** nodes and **spleen**. It undermines the immune system, leaving the sufferer susceptible to infection. However, it responds well to radiotherapy and **cytotoxic drugs**, and long-term survival is usual.

holistic medicine

In **alternative medicine**, umbrella term for an approach that virtually all alternative therapies profess, which considers the overall health and lifestyle profile of a patient, and treats specific ailments not primarily as conditions to be alleviated but rather as symptoms of more fundamental disease.

❝ A physician is obliged to consider more than a diseased organ, more even than the whole man – he must view the man in his world. ❞

Harvey Cushing, US surgeon, quoted in René' Dubos' *Man Adapting*.

homeopathy or homoeopathy

System of **alternative medicine** based on the principle that symptoms of disease are part of the body's self-healing processes, and on the practice of administering extremely diluted doses of natural substances found to produce in a healthy person the symptoms manifest in the illness being treated. Developed by the German physician Samuel Hahnemann (1755–1843), the system is increasingly practised today as an alternative to, or complementary to, allopathic (orthodox) medicine.

hormone

Chemical secretion of the ductless **endocrine glands**. The major glands are:

- the **thyroid**
- parathyroid
- **pituitary**
- adrenal
- **pancreas**
- **ovary**
- **testis**.

Historically, the first evidence of a hormone's existence has often been an unexplained disease which subsequently turns out to be caused by over- or under-secretion of the hormone. In recent years, hormonal imbalances have been implicated in the production of some forms of **cancer,** particularly cancer of the breast and uterus in women and of the prostate gland in men.

There are also hormone-secreting cells in:

- the kidney
- liver
- gastrointestinal tract
- thymus (in the neck)
- pineal (in the brain)
- placenta.

Many human diseases that are caused by hormone deficiency can be treated with hormone preparations. Hormones bring about changes in the functions of various organs according to the body's requirements. The hypothalamus, which adjoins the pituitary gland at the base of the brain, is a control centre for overall coordination of hormone secretion.

- The thyroid hormones determine the rate of general body chemistry;
- the adrenal hormones prepare the organism during stress for 'fight or flight' (see **anxiety**);
- the sexual hormones such as **oestrogen** and **testosterone** govern reproductive functions;
- hormones, such as **insulin** and aldosterone, are essential for life.

hormone replacement therapy (HRT)
Use of **oestrogen** and **progesterone** to help limit the unpleasant effects of the **menopause** in women. The treatment was first used in the 1970s. At the menopause, the ovaries cease to secrete natural oestrogen. This results in a number of symptoms, including hot flushes, anxiety, and a change in the pattern of menstrual bleeding. It is also associated with **osteoporosis**, or a thinning of bones, leading to an increased incidence of fractures. Oestrogen preparations, taken to replace the decline in natural hormone levels, combined with regular exercise can help to maintain bone strength in women. In order to improve bone density, however, HRT must be taken for five years, during which time the woman will continue to menstruate. Many women do not find this acceptable. In 1997 about 33% of British women and 40% of US women opted for post-menopausal HRT.

human body
The physical structure of the human being. It develops from the single **cell** of the fertilized ovum (egg), is born after 40 weeks' gestation (development between conception and birth), and usually reaches sexual maturity between 11 and 18 years of age. The bony framework (**skeleton**) consists of more than 200 bones, over half of which are in the hands and feet. Bones are held together by joints, some of which allow movement. The circulatory system supplies muscles and organs with **blood**, which provides oxygen and nourishment

and removes carbon dioxide and other waste products. Body functions are controlled by the **nervous system** and **hormones**. In the upper part of the trunk is the thorax, which contains the **lungs** and **heart**. Below this is the abdomen, containing the **digestive system** (stomach and intestines); the **liver**, **spleen**, and **pancreas**; the **urinary system** (kidneys, ureter, and bladder); and, in women, the reproductive organs (**ovaries**, **uterus**, and **vagina**). In men, the prostate gland and seminal vesicles are situated in the abdomen, the **testes** being in the scrotum, which, with the **penis**, is suspended in front of and below the abdomen. The bladder empties through a small channel (urethra); in the female this opens in the upper end of the vulval cleft, which also contains the opening of the vagina, or birth canal; in the male, the urethra is continued into the penis. In both sexes, the lower bowel terminates in the anus, a ring of strong muscle situated between the buttocks.

humerus
The long **bone** of the upper arm.

Huntington's chorea
Rare **hereditary** disease of the **nervous system** that mostly begins in middle age. It is characterized by involuntary movements (chorea), emotional disturbances, and rapid mental degeneration progressing to **dementia**. There is no known cure but the genetic mutation giving rise to the disease was located 1993, making it easier to test for the disease and increasing the chances of developing a cure in the future.

hydrocephalus
Potentially serious increase in the volume of cerebrospinal fluid (CSF) within the ventricles of the brain. In infants, since their skull plates have not fused, it causes enlargement of the head and there is a risk of brain damage from CSF pressure on the developing brain. Hydrocephalus may be due to mechanical obstruction of the outflow of CSF from the ventricles or to faulty reabsorption. It may occur as a consequence of brain injury or disease. Treatment usually

involves surgical placement of a shunt system to drain the fluid into the abdominal cavity. In infants, the condition is often seen in association with **spina bifida**.

hydrotherapy
In **alternative medicine**, use of water, externally or internally, for health or healing. Programmed hot and/or cold applications or immersions, sometimes accompanied by local low-voltage stimulation, are used to alleviate tension and stress. Some hydrotherapists specialize in colonic or high colonic irrigation, the thorough washing-out and detoxification of the **digestive system**.

hypertension
Abnormally high **blood pressure** due to a variety of causes, leading to excessive contraction of the smooth muscle cells of the walls of the arteries. It increases the risk of kidney disease, **stroke**, and **heart attack**. Hypertension is one of the major public health problems of the developed world, affecting between 15% and 20% of adults in industrialized countries (1996). It may be of unknown cause (essential hypertension), or it may occur in association with some other condition, such as kidney disease (secondary or symptomatic hypertension). It is controlled with a low-salt diet and drugs.

hyperthyroidism or thyrotoxicosis
Overactivity of the **thyroid** gland due to enlargement or **tumour**. Symptoms include accelerated heartbeat rate, sweating, anxiety, tremor, and weight loss. Treatment is by drugs or surgery.

hypochondria
Neurotic preoccupation with bodily functions and ill health. Hypochondriacs worry that they may be harbouring some kind of

❝ An imaginary ailment is worse than a disease. ❞

Yiddish proverb.

disease. In its severe form (hypochondriasis), which is usually due to underlying anxiety or depression, the patient harbours delusions of ill health.

hypothermia

Condition in which the deep (core) temperature of the body (see **body temerature**) falls below 35°C. If it is not discovered, **coma**, and death ensue. Most at risk are the elderly and babies (particularly if premature).

hypothyroidism or myxoedema

Deficient functioning of the **thyroid** gland, causing slowed mental and physical performance, weight gain, sensitivity to cold, and susceptibility to infection. This may be due to lack of iodine in the diet or a defect of the thyroid gland, both being productive of goitre; or to the **pituitary** gland providing insufficient stimulus to the thyroid gland. Treatment of thyroid deficiency is by the **hormone** thyroxine. When present from birth, untreated hypothyroidism can lead to cretinism.

hysterectomy

Surgical removal of all or part of the **uterus** (womb). The operation is performed to treat fibroids (benign **tumours** growing in the uterus) or **cancer**; it is sometimes carried out to relieve heavy menstrual bleeding. A woman who has had a hysterectomy will no longer menstruate and cannot bear children.

Instead of a full hysterectomy it is sometimes possible to remove the lining of the womb, the endometrium, by a 'keyhole' procedure known as endometrial resection, using either diathermy or a laser.

hysteria

According to the work of Sigmund Freud, the conversion of a psychological conflict or anxiety feeling into a physical symptom, such as paralysis, blindness, recurrent cough, vomiting, and general malaise. The term is little used today. The term is also used to describe a condition of extreme emotional excitement.

immunity

The protection the body has against foreign **micro-organisms**, such as **bacteria** and **viruses**, and against cancerous cells (see **cancer**). The cells that provide this protection are called **white blood cells**, or leucocytes, and make up the immune system. They include neutrophils and macrophages, which can engulf invading organisms and other unwanted material, and natural killer cells that destroy cells infected by viruses and cancerous cells. Some of the most important immune cells are the B cells and T cells. Immune cells coordinate their activities by means of chemical messengers or lymphokines, including the antiviral messenger interferon. The lymph nodes play a major role in organizing the immune response.

Immunity is also provided by a range of physical barriers such as the skin, tear fluid, acid in the stomach, and mucus in the airways. AIDS is one of many viral diseases in which the immune system is affected.

immunization

Conferring immunity to infectious disease by artificial methods. The most widely used technique is vaccination (see **vaccine**). Immunization is an important public health measure. If most of the population has been immunized against a particular disease, it is impossible for an epidemic to take hold.

Vaccination against **smallpox** was developed by Edward **Jenner** in 1796. In the late 19th century Louis **Pasteur** developed **vaccines** against cholera, typhoid, typhus, plague, and yellow fever.

immunosuppressive

Any drug that suppresses the body's normal immune responses to infection or foreign tissue. It is used in the treatment of autoimmune disease; as part of **chemotherapy** for **leukaemias**, lymphomas, and other cancers; and to help prevent rejection following organ **transplantation**. Immunosuppressed patients are at greatly increased risk of infection.

In March 1998 the US Food and Drug Administration (FDA) approved the drug Viagra for prescription to people who suffer from impotence. Viagra works by dilating the blood vessels of the penis and must be taken about an hour before intercourse. Side effects include headaches and fainting (due to dilation of blood vessels elsewhere), and blue tinted vision.

impetigo

Skin infection with either streptococcus or staphylococcus **bacteria**, characterized by encrusted yellow sores on the skin. Particularly common in infants and small children, it is highly contagious but curable with antibiotics.

impotence

Physical inability to perform sexual intercourse (the term is not usually applied to women). Impotent men fail to achieve an erection and this may be due to illness, the effects of certain drugs, or psychological factors.

incontinence

Failure or inability to control evacuation of the bladder or bowel (or both in the case of double incontinence). It may arise as a result of injury, childbirth, disease, or senility.

indigestion or dyspepsia

Any pain or discomfort in the stomach or abdomen due to problems in the **digestive system**.

> *Many people think they have religion when they are troubled with dyspepsia.*
>
> **Robert G Ingersoll**, *Liberty of Man, Woman and Child'*, Section 3.

infant mortality rate

Measure of the number of infants dying under one year of age, usually expressed as the number of deaths per 1,000 live births. Improved sanitation, nutrition, and medical care have considerably lowered figures throughout much of the world; for example in the 18th century in the USA and UK infant mortality was about 500 per thousand, compared with the current figure of 10 per thousand. In developing contries, however, the infant mortality rate remains high.

inflammation

Defensive reaction of the body tissues to disease or damage, including redness, swelling, and heat. Denoted by the suffix *-itis* (as in appendicitis), it may be acute or chronic and may be accompanied by the formation of **pus**. This is an essential part of the healing process. Inflammation occurs when damaged cells release a substance (histamine) that causes blood vessels to widen and leak into the surrounding tissues. This phenomenon accounts for the redness, swelling, and heat. Pain is due partly to the pressure of swelling and also to irritation of nerve endings. Defensive **white blood cells** congregate within an area of inflammation to engulf and remove foreign matter and dead tissue.

The 1918–19 influenza pandemic killed about 20 million people worldwide.

influenza

Any of various viral infections primarily affecting the air passages, accompanied by systemic effects such as **fever**, chills, headache, joint and muscle pains, and lassitude. Treatment is with bed rest and analgesic drugs such as **aspirin** or **paracetamol**. Depending on the virus strain, influenza varies in virulence and duration, and there is always the risk of secondary (bacterial) infection of the lungs (**pneumonia**). Vaccines are effective against known strains but will not give protection against newly evolving viruses.

insomnia
Difficulty in falling asleep and sustaining sleep. Insomnia may be caused by mental or physical factors, with **anxiety** being the commonest cause. It results in the sufferer feeling perpetually tired.

insulin
Hormone, produced by specialized cells in the islets of Langerhans in the **pancreas**, that regulates the **metabolism** (rate of activity) of glucose, fats, and proteins. Insulin was discovered by Canadian physician Frederick Banting and Canadian physiologist Charles Best, who pioneered its use in treating **diabetes**. Normally, insulin is secreted in response to rising blood sugar levels (after a meal, for example), stimulating the body's cells to store the excess. Failure of this regulatory mechanism in diabetes mellitus requires treatment with insulin injections or capsules taken by mouth. Types vary from pig and beef insulins to synthetic and bioengineered ones. They may be combined with other substances to make them longer- or shorter-acting.

intestine
The digestive tract from the stomach outlet to the anus. The small intestine is 6 m/20 ft long, 4 cm/1.5 in in diameter and consists of the duodenum, jejunum, and ileum; the large intestine is 1.5 m/5 ft long, 6 cm/2.5 in in diameter and includes the caecum, colon, and rectum. Both are muscular tubes comprising an inner lining that secretes alkaline digestive juice, a submucous coat containing fine blood vessels and nerves, a muscular coat, and a serous coat covering all, supported by a strong peritoneum, which carries the blood and lymph vessels and the nerves. The contents are passed along slowly by **peristalsis** (waves of involuntary muscular action).

intrauterine device (IUD) or coil

A **contraceptive** device that is inserted into the womb (**uterus**). It is a tiny plastic object, sometimes containing copper. By causing a mild **inflammation** of the lining of the uterus it prevents fertilized eggs from becoming implanted. IUDs are not usually given to women who have not had children. The device is generally very reliable, as long as it remains in place, with a success rate of about 98%. Some women experience heavier and more painful periods and there is a very slight risk of a pelvic infection leading to infertility.

in vitro fertilization (IVF)

Allowing eggs (ova) and sperm to unite in a laboratory to form **embryos**. The embryos (properly called pre-embryos in their two- to eight-celled state) are stored by cooling to the temperature of liquid air (cryopreservation) until they are implanted into the womb (uterus) of an otherwise infertile mother (an extension of artificial insemination). The first baby to be produced by this method was born in 1978 in the UK. In cases where the **Fallopian** tubes are blocked, fertilization may be carried out by intra-vaginal culture, in which egg and sperm are incubated (in a plastic tube) in the mother's vagina, then transferred surgically into the uterus. As yet the success rate is relatively low; only 15–20% of in vitro fertilizations result in live births.

iridology

Diagnostic technique in **alternative medicine** based on correspondences between specific areas of the iris of the eye and bodily functions and organs. It was discovered in the 19th century independently by a Hungarian and a Swedish physician and later refined and developed in the USA by Bernard Jensen. Iridology is of proven effectiveness in monitoring general wellbeing and indicating the presence of organic disorders but cannot be as specific about the nature and extent of these as orthodox diagnostic techniques.

irritable bowel syndrome
Condition characterized by episodes of lower abdominal pain with constipation or **diarrhoea**. The symptoms are caused by spasming of the colon but there is no underlying disease. The condition is often associated with stress or anxiety. It responds to antispasmodic drugs and measures to reduce stress.

jaundice

Yellow discoloration of the skin and whites of the eyes caused by an excess of bile pigment in the bloodstream. Approximately 60% of newborn babies exhibit some degree of jaundice, which is treated by bathing in white, blue, or green light that converts the bile pigment bilirubin into a water-soluble compound that can be excreted in urine. A serious form of jaundice occurs in rhesus disease (see **rhesus factor**). Bile pigment is normally produced by the **liver** from the breakdown of **red blood cells**, then excreted into the **intestines**. A buildup in the blood is due to abnormal destruction of red cells (as in some cases of **anaemia**), impaired liver function (as in **hepatitis**), or blockage in the excretory channels (as in gallstones or cirrhosis). The jaundice gradually recedes following treatment of the underlying cause.

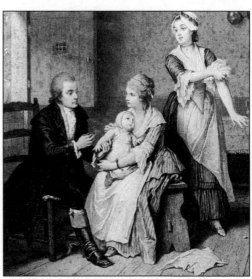

Jenner, Edward
(1749–1823)

English physician who pioneered vaccination (see **immunization** and **vaccine**). His discovery in 1796 that inoculation with cowpox gives immunity to **smallpox**, then a major killer, was a great medical break-

Jenner *19th-century woodcut showing Edward Jenner administering the first-ever smallpox vaccination on 14 May 1796 on the 8 year old James Phipps.*

through. Jenner observed that people who worked with cattle and contracted cowpox from them never subsequently caught smallpox. In 1798 he published his findings that a child inoculated with cowpox, then two months later with smallpox, did not get smallpox. He coined the word 'vaccination' from the Latin word for cowpox, *vaccinia*. Jenner was born in Berkeley,

In 1788, an epidemic of smallpox swept Gloucestershire and inoculations with live vaccine, taken from a person with a mild attack of the disease, were used. This method had been brought to England from Turkey in 1721 by Lady Mary Wortley Montagu and further developed by Dutch physiolgist Jan Ingerhousz. It was during this epidemic that Jenner made his initial observations.

Gloucestershire, and studied at St George's Hospital, London. Returning to Berkeley, he set up a medical practice there.

jet lag

The effect of a sudden switch of time zones in air travel, resulting in tiredness and feeling 'out of step' with day and night. It has been suggested that use of the **hormone** melatonin helps to lessen the effect of jet lag by resetting the body clock.

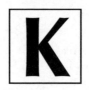

keratin
Fibrous protein found in the skin of vertebrates and also in hair and nails. If pressure is put on some parts of the **skin**, more keratin is produced, forming thick calluses that protect the layers of skin beneath.

keyhole surgery
(Or minimally invasive surgery) Term used to describe operations that do not involve cutting into the body in the traditional way (open surgery). Procedures are performed either by means of **endoscopy** or by passing fine instruments through catheters inserted into the body by way of large blood vessels. Probably the best-known example is percutaneous transluminal coronary angioplasty (PTCA) to treat **coronary artery disease**. It involves passing a balloon-tipped catheter into a large artery in the groin and advancing it until the tip comes to rest in a narrowed coronary vessel; the balloon is then inflated to widen the diseased vessel. PTCA is performed in selected cases as an alternative to the conventional procedure of coronary artery bypass grafting (CABG). Advocates of keyhole surgery claim it is safer and cheaper than conventional surgery, requiring a shorter hospital stay. However, one or two such procedures have been called into question, either because they do not yield the long-term result of open surgery or because they are performed by people inexperienced in the technique. In roughly a third of cases treated by PTCA, for instance, the artery becomes blocked again within six months, requiring further surgery.

kidney
One of a pair of organs responsible for fluid regulation, excretion of waste products, and maintaining the chemical composition of the blood. The kidneys are situated on the rear wall of the abdomen. Each

one consists of a number of long tubules; the outer parts filter the aqueous components of blood and the inner parts selectively reabsorb vital salts, leaving waste products in the remaining fluid (urine), which is passed through the ureter to the bladder (see **urinary system**). If one kidney is removed, the other enlarges to take over its function. A patient with two defective kidneys may continue near-normal life with the aid of **dialysis**; or a kidney **transplant** may be recommended. Diseases of the kidney include the formation of kidney stones. These hard stones can build up as a result of high levels of blood calcium or uric acid, and can cause intense pain as they travel down the ureter, with bleeding in the urinary tract.

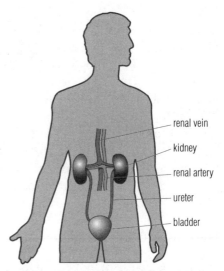

kidney *Blood enters the kidney through the renal artery. The blood is filtered through the glomeruli to extract the nitrogenous waste products and excess water that make up urine. The urine flows through the ureter to the bladder; the cleaned blood then leaves the kidney via the renal vein.*

Koch, (Heinrich Hermann) Robert
(1843–1910)
German bacteriologist. Koch and his assistants devised the techniques for culturing **bacteria** outside the body and formulated the rules for

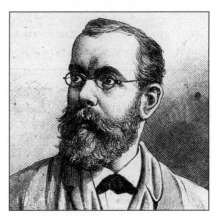

Koch *Robert Koch, German bacteriologist who identified the bacteria responsible for tuberculosis and cholera.*

showing whether or not a bacterium is the cause of a disease. He was awarded the Nobel Prize for Physiology or Medicine in 1905. His techniques enabled him to identify the bacteria responsible for

Koch also showed that rats are vectors (carriers) of bubonic plague and that sleeping sickness is transmitted by the tsetse fly.

tuberculosis (1882), cholera (1883) and other diseases. He investigated anthrax bacteria in the 1870s and showed that they form spores which spread the infection. Koch was born near Hannover and studied at Göttingen. He was professor at Berlin duing 1885–91, when he became director of the newly established Institute for Infectious Diseases, but he resigned in 1904 and spent much of the rest of his life advising other countries on ways to combat various diseases.

Krebs, Hans Adolf (1900–1981)
German-born British biochemist. In 1953 he shared the Nobel Prize for Physiology or medicine for the discovery of the citric acid cycle, now known as the Krebs' cycle, by which food is converted to energy in living tissues.

labour
The sequence of events in childbirth, from the first contraction of the womb through to delivery. There are three stages of labour, normally spread over some hours.

lacrimal apparatus
Apparatus that supplies and drains the fluid needed to lubricate and cleanse the surface of the **eye**. The lacrimal gland in the upper eyelid secretes this fluid, which in quantity is known as tears; it drains through a tiny opening in the inner corner of the eye into the lacrimal canaliculus and from there passes into the nasal cavity by way of the nasolacrimal duct.

Landsteiner, Karl (1868–1943)
Austrian-born immunologist who discovered the ABO **blood group** system during 1900 and 1902 and aided in the discovery of the **Rhesus blood factors** in 1940. Whilst working in the USA, he also discovered the **polio** virus. He was awarded the Nobel Prize for Physiology or Medicine in 1930.

laryngitis
Inflammation of the larynx, causing soreness of the throat, a dry cough, and hoarseness. The acute form is due to a **virus** or other infection, excessive use of the voice, or inhalation of irritating smoke, and may cause the voice to be completely lost. With rest, the inflammation usually subsides in a few days.

laser surgery
Use of intense light sources to cut, coagulate, or vaporize tissue. Less invasive than normal surgery, the procedure destroys diseased

tissue gently and allows quicker, more natural healing. It can be used by way of a flexible **endoscope** to enable the surgeon to view the diseased area at which the laser needs to be aimed.

laxative

Substance used to relieve constipation (infrequent bowel movement). Current medical opinion discourages regular or prolonged use of laxatives. Regular exercise and a diet high in vegetable fibre are believed to be the best means of preventing and treating constipation.

> 6 The confidence and security of a people can be measured by their attitude towards laxatives. 9
>
> **Florence King**, US writer, *Reflections in a Jaundiced Eye.*

Leeuwenhoek, Anton van (1632–1723)

Dutch draper who pioneered microscopic research. He ground his own lenses, some of which magnified up to 200 times. With these he was able to distinguish individual **red blood cells**, **sperm**, and **bacteria**, achievements which no one was able to repeat for more than a century.

legionnaires' disease

Pneumonia-like disease, so called because it was first identified when it broke out at a convention of the American Legion in Philadelphia in 1976. Legionnaires' disease is caused by the bacterium *Legionella pneumophila*, which breeds in warm water (for example, in the cooling towers of air-conditioning systems). It is spread in minute water droplets, which may be inhaled. The disease can be treated successfully with **antibiotics**, though mortality can be high in elderly patients.

leprosy or Hansen's disease

Chronic, progressive disease caused by a bacterium *Mycobacterium leprae* closely related to that of **tuberculosis**. The infection attacks the skin and nerves. Once common in many countries, leprosy is now confined almost entirely to the tropics. It is controlled with drugs. In 1998 there were an estimated

In January 1998 the Indian government authorized the sale of the world's first leprosy **vaccine**. It is effective for only 6–12 months.

1.5 million cases of leprosy, with 60% of these being in India. The visible effects of long-standing leprosy (joint damage, paralysis, and loss of fingers or toes) are due to nerve damage and injuries of which the sufferer may be unaware. Damage to the nerves remains, and the technique of using the patient's muscle material to encourage nerve regrowth is being explored.

leucocyte
Another name for a **white blood cell**.

leukaemia
Any one of a group of **cancers** of the blood cells, with widespread involvement of the bone marrow and other blood-forming tissue. The central feature of leukaemia is runaway production of **white blood cells** that are immature or in some way abnormal. These rogue cells, which lack the defensive capacity of healthy white cells, overwhelm the normal ones, leaving the victim vulnerable to infection. Treatment is with **radiotherapy** and **cytotoxic** drugs to suppress replication of abnormal cells, or by bone-marrow transplantation. Abnormal functioning of the bone marrow also suppresses production of **red blood cells** and blood platelets, resulting in **anaemia** and a failure of the blood to clot. Leukaemias are classified into acute or chronic, depending on their known rates of progression. They are also grouped according to the type of white cell involved.

libido
Sexual drive. Loss of libido is seen in some diseases.
   See also: *impotence.*

life expectancy

Average lifespan that can be presumed of a person at birth. It depends on nutrition, disease control, environmental contaminants, war, stress, and living standards in general. There is a marked difference between industrialized countries, which generally have an ageing population, and the poorest countries, where life expectancy is much shorter:

- in Bangladesh, life expectancy is currently 48 years;
- in Nigeria it is 49 years;
- in famine-prone Ethiopia only 41 years;
- in the UK, average life expectancy currently stands at 74 years for males and about 80 years for females.

Lister, Joseph (1827–1912)

English surgeon. He was the founder of antiseptic surgery, influenced by Louis **Pasteur's** work on **bacteria**. He introduced the application of dressings soaked in carbolic acid and established strict rules of hygiene to combat wound sepsis in hospitals.

Learning of Pasteur's discovery of **micro-organisms**, however, Lister began to use carbolic acid as a disinfectant. In 1867 he announced that his wards in the Glasgow Royal Infirmary in Scotland had remained clear of sepsis for nine months. Later he adopted the method developed by Robert **Koch** in

Lister *A 19th-century portrait of Joseph Lister, the founder of antiseptic surgery.*

Germany of using steam to sterilize surgical instruments and dressings. The number of surgical operations had greatly increased following the introduction of **anaesthetics** but death rates were more than 40%. Under Lister's regime fatalities after surgery fell dramatically.

Lister was born in Upton, Essex, and studied at University College, London. He was professor of surgery at Glasgow 1860–69, at Edinburgh 1869–77, and at King's College, London, 1877–92.

liver
Large organ which has many regulatory and storage functions. The human liver is situated in the upper abdomen and weighs about 2 kg/4.5 lb. It is divided into four lobes. The liver receives the products of digestion (see **digestive system**), converts glucose to glycogen (a long-chain **carbohydrate** used for storage), and then back to glucose when needed. In this way the liver regulates the level of glucose in the blood. It removes excess amino acids from the blood, converting them to urea, which is excreted by the **kidneys**. The liver also synthesizes vitamins, produces bile and blood-clotting factors, and removes damaged red cells and **toxins** such as **alcohol** from the blood.

living will
Written declaration of a person's wishes regarding medical treatment if in the future he or she should become too ill to communicate. It is in effect an advance refusal of heroic interventions to prolong a life that the patient would consider no longer tolerable. It enables patients whose condition is terminal to die with dignity. Living wills are increasingly popular in the USA.

lumbago
Pain in the lower region of the back, usually due to strain or faulty posture. If it occurs with **sciatica**, it may be due to pressure on spinal nerves by a **slipped disc**. Treatment includes rest, application of heat, and skilled manipulation. Surgery may be needed in rare cases. Lumbago is typically sudden in onset, with an acute pain afflicting the person during some movement of the back. In some cases the onset of pain is gradual and becomes increasingly severe. The lumbar muscles go into spasmodic contraction.

lumbar puncture or spinal tap

Insertion of a hollow needle between two lumbar (lower back) **vertebrae** to withdraw a sample of cerebrospinal fluid (CSF) for testing and diagnosis. Normally clear and colourless, the CSF acts as a fluid buffer around the brain and spinal cord. Changes in its quantity, colour, or composition may indicate neurological damage or disease.

lung

One of two large organs in the chest used for gas exchange. It is essentially a sheet of thin, moist membrane that is folded so as to

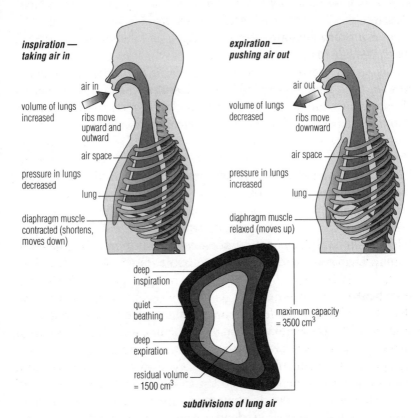

lung *The role of the lungs in respiration. Gas exchange occurs in the alveoli, tiny air tubes in the lungs.*

occupy less space. The lung tissue, consisting of multitudes of air sacs (alveoli) and blood vessels, is very light and spongy, and functions by bringing inhaled air into close contact with the blood so that oxygen can pass in and waste carbon dioxide can be passed out. The efficiency of lungs is enhanced by breathing movements, by the thinness and moistness of their surfaces, and by a constant supply of circulating blood. Air is drawn into the lungs through the trachea and bronchi by the expansion of the ribs and the contraction of the diaphragm. The principal diseases of the lungs are **tuberculosis**, **pneumonia**, **bronchitis**, **emphysema**, and **cancer**.

lupus

Any of various diseases characterized by lesions of the **skin**. One form (lupus vulgaris) is caused by the tubercle bacillus (see **tuberculosis**). The organism produces **ulcers** that spread and eat away the underlying tissues. Treatment is primarily with standard antituberculous drugs but ultraviolet light may also be used. Lupus erythematosus (LE) has two forms: discoid LE, seen as red, scaly patches on the skin, especially the face; and disseminated or systemic LE, which may affect connective tissue anywhere in the body, often involving the internal organs. The latter is much more serious. Treatment is with **corticosteroids**. LE is an autoimmune disease.

lymph

Fluid found in the lymphatic system. It is drained from the tissues by lymph capillaries, which empty into larger lymph vessels (lymphatics). These lead to lymph nodes (small, round bodies chiefly situated in the neck, armpit, groin, thorax, and abdomen), which process the lymphocytes (type of **white blood cells**) produced by the bone marrow and filter out harmful substances and **bacteria**. From the lymph nodes, vessels carry the lymph to the thoracic duct and the right lymphatic duct, which drain into the large veins in the neck. Lymph carries some nutrients and white blood cells to the tissues, and waste matter away from them. It exudes from capillaries into the tissue spaces between the cells and is similar in composition to blood **plasma**.

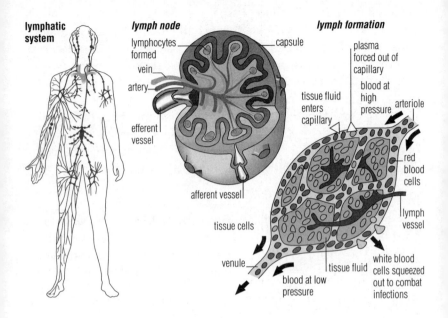

lymphatic system

lymph node

lymphocytes formed

vein

artery

efferent vessel

capsule

afferent vessel

tissue cells

venule

blood at low pressure

lymph formation

plasma forced out of capillary

blood at high pressure

tissue fluid enters capillary

arteriole

red blood cells

lymph vessel

tissue fluid

white blood cells squeezed out to combat infections

lymph *The lymph vessels form a network called the lymphatic system. At various points in the lymphatic system, lymph nodes filter and clean the lymph.*

magnetic resonance imaging (MRI)

Diagnostic **scanning** system based on the principles of nuclear magnetic resonance. MRI yields finely detailed three-dimensional images of structures within the body without exposing the patient to harmful radiation (which is a hazard of using X-rays). The technique is invaluable for imaging the soft tissues of the body, in particular the brain and the spinal cord. Claimed as the biggest breakthrough in diagnostic imaging since the discovery of X-rays, MRI is a

Also developed around magnetic technology, magnetic resonance spectroscopy (MRS) is a technique for investigating conditions in which there is a disturbance of the body's energy metabolism, including ischaemia and toxic damage due to drugs or other chemicals. MRS is also of value in diagnosing some cancers.

noninvasive technique based on a magnet which is many thousands of times stronger than the Earth's magnetic field. It causes nuclei within the atoms of the body to align themselves in one direction. When a brief radio pulse is beamed at the body the nuclei spin, emitting weak radio signals as they realign themselves to the magnet. These signals, which are characteristic for each type of tissue, are converted electronically into images on a viewing screen.

malaria

Infectious parasitic disease of the tropics transmitted by mosquitoes, marked by periodic fever and an enlarged **spleen**. When a female mosquito of the *Anopheles* genus bites a person who has malaria, it

Some half a billion people worldwide suffer periodic attacks of malaria and the disease claims an estimated two million lives each year.

malaria *The life cycle of the malaria parasite is split between mosquito and human hosts. The parasites are injected into the human bloodstream by an infected* Anopheles *mosquito and carried to the liver. Here the parasites attack red blood cells, and multiply asexually. The infected blood cells burst, producing spores, or merozoites, which reinfect the bloodstream. After several generations, the parasite develops into a sexual form. If the human host is bitten at this stage, the sexual form of the parasite is sucked into the mosquito's stomach. Here fertilization takes place, the zygotes formed reproduce asexually and migrate to the salivary glands ready to be injected into another human host, completing the cycle.*

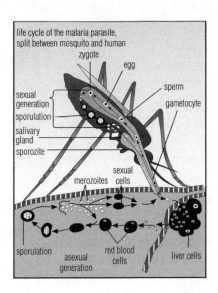

ingests, along with the victim's blood, one of four malaria protozoa of the genus *Plasmodium*. This matures within the insect and is then transferred when the mosquito bites a new victim.

Quinine, the first drug used against malaria, has now been replaced by synthetic drugs. However, resistant strains of the main malaria parasite, *Plasmodium fulciparum*, are spreading rapidly in many parts of the world.

malnutrition

Condition resulting from a defective diet where certain important food elements (such as **proteins**, **vitamins**, or **carbohydrates**) are absent. It can lead to deficiency diseases. A related problem is undernourishment.

See also: *nutrition*.

A high global death rate linked to malnutrition has arisen from famine situations caused by global warming, droughts, and the greenhouse effect as well as by sociopolitical factors such as alcohol and drug abuse, poverty and war. In 1998 there was an estimated 180 million malnourished children worldwide.

mammography
X-ray procedure used to screen for breast **cancer**. An important health screening test, it can detect abnormal growths at an early stage, before they can be seen with the eye, or detected manually.

manic depression or bipolar disorder
Mental disorder characterized by recurring periods of either depression or mania (inappropriate elation, agitation, and rapid thought and speech) or both. Sufferers may be genetically predisposed to the condition. Some cases have been improved by taking prescribed doses of lithium. Some manic-depressive patients have only manic attacks, others only depressive, and in others the alternating, or circular, form exists. The episodes may be of varying severity, from mild to **psychotic** (when the patient loses touch with reality and may experience **hallucinations**), and may sometimes continue for years without interruption.

marijuana
Dried leaves and flowers of the hemp plant cannabis, used as a drug; it is illegal in most countries. It is eaten or inhaled and causes euphoria, distortion of time, and heightened sensations of sight and sound. Mexico is the world's largest producer.

- A report released in March 1999 by the Institute of Medicine in the USA said that marijuana should be subjected to clinical tests because it helps fight pain and nausea.

- A US study involving 3,882 people who had survived heart attacks revealed that smoking marijuana may increase the risk of a heart attack, by as much as five times for an hour after smoking. The risk may increase because marijuana increases the heart rate by about 40 beats a minute.

- In 1999 research began into the beneficial effects of marijuana in cases of MS (**multiple sclerosis**).

massage

Manipulation of the soft tissues of the body, the muscles, ligaments, and tendons, either to encourage the healing of specific injuries or to produce the general beneficial effects of relaxing muscular tension, stimulating blood circulation, and improving the tone and strength of the skin and muscles.

The benefits of massage were known to the ancient Chinese, Egyptian, and Greek cultures. The techniques most widely practised today were developed by the Swedish physician Per Henrik Ling (1776–1838).

mastectomy

Surgical removal of a breast. Performed for **cancer**, it may also involve removal of lymphatic tissue in the armpit. A double masectomy refers to the removal of both breasts.

ME

Abbreviation for myalgic encephalomyelitis, a debilitating condition still not universally accepted as a genuine disease. The condition occurs after a flulike episode and has a diffuse range of symptoms. These strike and recur for years and include extreme fatigue, muscular pain, weakness, poor balance and coordination, joint pains, gastric upset, and depression. It is sometimes known as postviral syndrome or chronic fatigue syndrome. There is no definitive treatment for ME but over time the symptoms become less severe.

measles

Acute virus disease (rubeola), spread by airborne infection. Symptoms are fever, severe **catarrh**, small spots inside the mouth, and a raised, blotchy red rash visible for about a week after two weeks' incubation. Prevention is by vaccination. In industrialized countries it is not usually a serious disease, though serious complications may ensue and many deaths occur among children of developing countries. The North and South American Indians died by the thousands in measles epidemics of the 17th, 18th, and 19th centuries. In the UK the combined **MMR vaccine**, which protects against measles, mumps, and rubella (German measles), has proved very effective.

> ❝ They say love's like measles – all the worse when it comes late in life. ❞
>
> **Douglas Jerrold**, *Wit and Opinions of Douglas Jerrold, A Philanthropist.*

Medawar, Sir Peter Brian (1915–1987)

British zoologist who discovered acquired immune tolerance when he found that mature animals who have been injected with foreign cells early in life accept skin grafts from the original donor. He was awarded the 1960 Nobel Prize in Physiology or Medicine, jointly with Sir Frank Macfarlane Burnet, for his work on immunology.

See also: *immunity.*

melanin

Brown pigment that gives colour to the eyes, skin, hair, feathers, and scales of many vertebrates. In humans, melanin helps protect the skin against ultraviolet radiation from sunlight. Both genetic and environmental factors determine the amount of melanin in the skin.

Mendel, Gregor Johann (1822–1884)

Austrian biologist, founder of genetics. His experiments with successive generations of peas gave the basis for his theory of

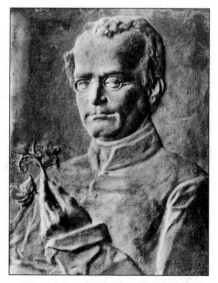

Mendel *A stone relief of Gregor Mendel, the founder of genetics.*

particulate inheritance. His results, published 1865–69, remained unrecognized for more than 30 years. Mendel concluded that each parent plant contributes a 'factor' to its offspring that determines a particular trait and that the pairs of factors in the offspring do not give rise to a blend of traits. Much of his work was performed on the edible pea *Pisum,* which he grew in his monastery garden. He carefully self-pollinated and wrapped (to prevent accidental pollination by insects) each individual plant, col-

Sub-Saharan Africa is known as the 'meningitis belt', with an incidence of the disease 10 times that of Europe and the USA (50 cases per 100,000 people).

lected the seeds and studied the offspring of these seeds. Seeing that some plants bred true and others not, he worked out the pattern of inheritance of various traits. Mendel entered the Augustinian monastery in what is now Brno, in the Czech Republic, in 1843. Later he studied at Vienna. In 1868 he became abbot of the monastery.

Ménière's disease or Ménière's syndrome
Recurring condition of the inner **ear** caused by an accumulation of fluid in the labyrinth of the ear that affects mechanisms of both hearing and balance. It usually develops in the middle or later years. Symptoms, which include deafness, ringing in the ears (**tinnitus**), nausea, **vertigo**, and loss of balance, may be eased by drugs, but there is no cure. The vertigo and associated nausea of Ménière's disease are often difficult to treat. **Antihistamines** are effective in some patients. Surgical decompression of the fluid may relieve vertigo and prevent the condition worsening.

meningitis
Inflammation of the meninges (membranes) surrounding the brain, caused by bacterial or viral infection. Bacterial meningitis, though treatable by **antibiotics**, is a much more serious disease. Symptoms include fever, headache, nausea, neck stiffness, **delirium**, and

(rarely) **convulsions**.

Bacterial meningitis is caused by a number of pathogens, principally *Neisseria meningitidis*, a bacterium that colonizes the lining of the throat and is carried by 2–10% of the healthy population. Life-threatening illness results if the bacterium enters the bloodstream. There are three strains of bacterial meningitis: serogroups A, B, and C. **Vaccines** exist only for A and C. However, they do not provide long-term protection nor are they suitable for children under the age of two. B is the most prevalent of the groups, causing over 50% of cases in Europe and the USA. Many common viruses can cause the occasional case of meningitis, although usually in a relatively mild form. The treatment for viral meningitis is rest.

menopause

In women, the cessation of reproductive ability, characterized by menstruation (see **menstrual cycle**) becoming irregular and eventually ceasing. Its onset occurs most commonly at about the age of 50, but varies greatly. Menopause is usually uneventful, but some women suffer from complications such as flushing, (increaped temperature and reddening of the skin), excessive vaginal bleeding, and nervous disorders. Since the 1950s, hormone-replacement therapy (**HRT**), using **oestrogen** alone or with progestogen, a synthetic form of **progesterone**, has been developed to counteract such effects. Long-term use of HRT has been associated with an increased risk of certain cancers, and of clot formation in the blood vessels (**thrombosis**), but it is thought to reduce the risk of **osteoporosis** (thinning of the bones) leading to broken bones, which may be indirectly fatal, particularly in the elderly. The menopause is also known as the 'change of life'.

menstrual cycle

Cycle that occurs in females of reproductive age (see **puberty**) in which the body is prepared for **pregnancy**. At the beginning of the cycle, a Graafian (egg) follicle develops in the **ovary** and the inner wall of the **uterus** forms a soft, spongy lining. The egg is released from the ovary and the uterus lining (endometrium) becomes vascularized (filled with blood vessels). If fertilization does not occur, the

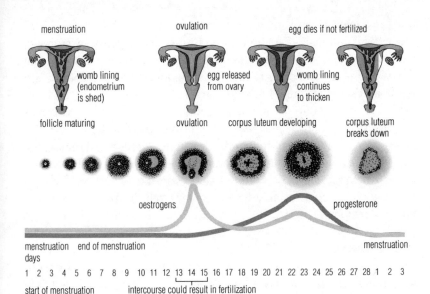

menstruation

ovulation

egg dies if not fertilized

womb lining
(endometrium
is shed)

egg released
from ovary

womb lining
continues
to thicken

follicle maturing

ovulation

corpus luteum developing

corpus luteum
breaks down

oestrogens

progesterone

menstruation   end of menstruation

menstruation

days

1 2 3 4 5 6 7 8 9 10 11 12 13 14 15 16 17 18 19 20 21 22 23 24 25 26 27 28 1 2 3

start of menstruation   intercourse could result in fertilization

menstrual cycle *From puberty to the menopause, most women produce a regular rhythm of hormones that stimulate the various stages of the menstrual cycle. The change in hormone levels may cause premenstrual tension. This diagram shows an average menstrual cycle. The dates of each stage vary from woman to woman.*

corpus luteum (remains of the Graafian follicle) degenerates; the uterine lining breaks down and is shed. This is what causes the loss of blood (commonly known as a period) that marks menstruation. The cycle then begins again. Menstruation takes place from puberty to **menopause**, except during pregnancy, occurring about every 28 days. The cycle is controlled by a number of **hormones**, including **oestrogen** and **progesterone**. If fertilization occurs, the corpus luteum persists and goes on producing progesterone.

metabolism

The chemical processes of living organisms enabling them to grow and to function. It involves a constant alternation of building up complex molecules (anabolism) and breaking them down (catabolism). For example, the process of digestion partially breaks down complex organic substances, ingested as food, which are subsequently resynthesized for use in the body (see **digestive system**). Within cells, complex molecules are broken down by the process of respiration (see **breathing**). The waste products of metabolism are removed by excretion.

metastasis
Spread of a malignant **tumour** from its original site. During metastasis, tumour cells become detached and enter blood or lymphatic vessels, travelling to other parts of the body.

micro-organism or microbe
Living organism invisible to the naked eye but visible under a microscope. Micro-organisms include **viruses** and single-celled organisms such as **bacteria**, protozoa, yeasts, and some algae. The study of micro-organisms is known as microbiology.

microsurgery
Part or all of an intricate surgical operation – rejoining a severed limb, for example – performed with the aid of a binocular microscope, using miniaturized instruments. Sewing of the nerves and blood vessels is done with a nylon thread so fine that it is only just visible to the naked eye. The technique permits treatment of previously inaccessible lesions in the eye or brain.

migraine
Acute, sometimes incapacitating headache (generally only on one side), accompanied by nausea, that recurs, often with advance symptoms such as visual disturbances. No cure has been discovered but anti-migraine drugs (such as ergotamine) normally relieve the symptoms. Some sufferers learn to avoid certain foods, such as chocolate, which suggests an

Belgian researchers trialled **vitamin** B2 successfully as a preventative for migraine, in 1998. The trial group took 400 mg doses of vitamin B2 daily and 59% of them experienced a halving or more in their headache frequency.

allergic factor (see **allergy**). The bacterium *Helicobacter pylori* has been linked to migraine by Italian researchers who found, in 1998, that 48% of migraine sufferers harboured the bacterium and that their migraine symptoms were greatly alleviated following **antibiotics** to eradicate *H. pylori*.

miscarriage

Spontaneous expulsion of a **fetus** from the womb before it is capable of independent survival. Miscarriage is believed to occur in 15% of pregnancies. Possible causes include fetal abnormality, abnormality of the **uterus** or **cervix**, infection, **shock**, underactive **thyroid**, and cocaine use.

MMR vaccine

Abbreviation for the combined **vaccine** given to small children to prevent **measles**, **mumps**, and rubella (**German measles**). There was a controversy over the use of this combined vaccine in early 1998, owing to the claims of a UK paediatrician that there was a slight risk of immunized children developing **autism**. This risk was deemed not to be present when the vaccinations were given as three separate shots at different times. Following this controversy, fewer British children were vaccinated; subsequent research has failed to substantiate the link.

mole or naevus

Patch of discoloration on the skin that has been present from birth. There are many different types of naevi, including those composed of a cluster of small blood vessels, such as the 'strawberry mark' (which usually disappears early in life) and the 'port-wine stain'. A mole of moderate size is harmless, and such marks can usually be disguised cosmetically unless they are extremely disfiguring, when they can sometimes be removed by cutting out, burning with an electric needle, freezing with carbon dioxide snow, or by argon laser treatment. In rare cases a mole may be a precursor of a malignant melanoma. Any changes in a mole, such as enlargement, itching, soreness, or bleeding, should be reported to a doctor.

morning sickness
Nausea and vomiting occurring mainly in the mornings during early **pregnancy**.

morphine
Narcotic alkaloid derived from opium and prescribed to alleviate severe pain. Its use produces serious side effects, including nausea, constipation, tolerance, and addiction, but it is highly valued for the relief of pain in the terminally ill. It is a controlled substance in many countries.

Morton, William Thomas Green (1819–1868)
US dentist who in 1846 introduced the use of ether as an **anaesthetic**. His claim to have been the first to do so was strongly disputed.

motion sickness
Nausea and vomiting caused by the motion of cars, boats, or other forms of transport. Constant vibration and movement sometimes stimulate changes in the fluid of the semicircular canals the inner **ear** (responsible for balance), to which the individual fails to adapt, and to which are added visual and psychological factors.

motor neurone disease (MND)
Chronic disease in which there is progressive degeneration of the **nerve cells** which instigate movement. It leads to weakness, wasting, and loss of **muscle** function and usually proves fatal within two to three years of onset. Motor neurone disease occurs in both familial and sporadic forms but its causes remain unclear. A **gene** believed to be implicated in familial cases was discovered in 1993.

Results of a US trial in 1995 showed that the drug myotrophin, a genetically engineered version of a chemical produced in the muscles, slowed deterioration in people with MND by 25%.

mucous membrane

Thin skin lining all body cavities and canals that come into contact with the air (for example, eyelids, breathing and digestive passages, and genital tract). It secretes **mucus**, a moistening, lubricating, and protective fluid.

mucus

Lubricating and protective fluid secreted by **mucous membranes** in many different parts of the body. In the gut, mucus smoothes the passage of food and keeps potentially damaging digestive enzymes away from the gut lining. In the lungs, it traps airborne particles so that they can be expelled.

multiple sclerosis (MS) or disseminated sclerosis

Incurable chronic disease of the **central nervous system** occurring in young or middle adulthood. Most prevalent in temperate zones, it affects more women than men. It is characterized by degeneration of the myelin sheath that surrounds nerves in the **brain** and **spinal cord**. Depending on where the demyelination occurs – which nerves are affected – the symptoms of MS can mimic almost any neurological disorder.

In the UK in December 1999 the Medical Research Council approved a three-year study to assess the benefits of **marijuana** in alleviating some of the symptoms of multiple sclerosis.

Typically seen are unsteadiness, ataxia (loss of muscular coordination), weakness, speech difficulties, and rapid involuntary movements of the eyes. The course of the disease is episodic, with

❝ Have you tried cannabis? I have heard it's the best thing for it. ❞

Charles, Prince of Wales, heir to the throne of Great Britain and Northern Ireland, talking to multiple sclerosis sufferer Karen Drake at the Sue Ryder Home in Cheltenham, *Daily Telegraph*, 24 December 1998.

frequent intervals of remission. Its cause is unknown but it may be initiated in childhood by some environmental factor, such as infection, in genetically susceptible people. In 1993 interferon beta 1b became the first drug to be approved in the USA for treating MS. It reduces the number and severity of relapses and slows the formation of brain lesions giving hope that it may slow down the progression of the disease.

mumps or infectious parotitis
Virus infection marked by fever, pain, and swelling of one or both parotid salivary glands (situated in front of the ears). It is usually shortlived in children, although **meningitis** is a possible complication. In adults the symptoms are more serious and it may cause sterility in men. Mumps is the most common cause of meningitis in children, but it follows a much milder course than bacterial meningitis and a complete recovery is usual. Rarely, mumps meningitis may lead to deafness. An effective **vaccine** against mumps, **measles,** and rubella (**MMR vaccine**) is now offered for children aged between 12 and 15 months.

muscle
Contractile tissue that produces locomotion and power. Muscle is made of long cells that can contract to between one-half and one-third of their relaxed length.
- Striped (or striated) muscles are activated by motor nerves under voluntary control; their ends are usually attached via **tendons** to **bones**. Striated muscle cells comprise the bulk of the musculature (about 40% of total body weight). Striated muscle is also known as striped, skeletal, somatic, or voluntary muscle.
- Involuntary or smooth muscles are controlled by motor nerves of the autonomic **nervous system** and are located in the gut, blood vessels, iris, and various ducts. Smooth muscle is found mostly in the walls of hollow viscera such as the **intestines** and its continuous contractions provide the motive power for digestion, secretion, and excretion. Smooth muscle is not under voluntary control.

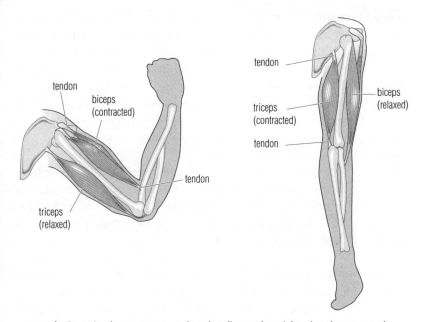

muscle *Even simple movements such as bending and straightening the arm require muscle pairs to contract and relax synchronously.*

- Cardiac muscle, which occurs only in the **heart**, is also controlled by the autonomic nervous system. Unlike somatic muscle fibres, its fibres branch so that the mass of muscle tends to function as one unit. Cardiac muscle continues to contract rhythmically when its nerve supply is cut.

A single nerve cell and all the muscle fibres which it innervates are collectively known as a motor unit. Where fine gradations of muscular activity are required, as with the muscles of the eyeball, motor units are small, perhaps comprising only one or two muscle fibres. On the other hand, powerful limb muscles need only relatively coarse control and a motor unit may include over a hundred muscle fibres.

In 1996, two US dentists discovered the existence of a muscle running from the jaw to just behind the eye socket. It is about 3cm/1in long and helps to support and raise the jaw.

A healthy muscle at rest is said to exhibit muscle tone, a firm feel, and characteristic elastic resistance to pressure. If the nerve supply to the muscle is cut, the muscle is paralyzed.

muscular dystrophy

Any of a group of inherited chronic **muscle** disorders marked by weakening and wasting of muscle. Muscle fibres degenerate, to be replaced by fatty tissue, although the nerve supply remains unimpaired. Death occurs in early adult life. The commonest form, 'Duchenne' muscular dystrophy, strikes boys (1 in 3,000), usually before the age of four. The child develops a waddling gait and an inward curvature (lordosis) of the lumbar spine. The muscles affected by dystrophy and the rate of progress vary. There is no cure, but physical treatments can minimize disability. Death usually occurs before the age of 20.

myasthenia gravis

An uncommon condition characterized by loss of **muscle** power, especially in the face and neck. The muscles tire rapidly and fail to respond to repeated nervous stimulation. Autoimmunity is the cause.

myocardial infarction

Medical term for a **heart attack**.

myopia or short-sightedness

Defect of the **eye** in which a person can see clearly only those objects that are close up. It is caused either by the eyeball being too long or by the cornea and lens system of the eye being too powerful, both of which cause the images of distant objects to be formed in front of the retina instead of on it. Nearby objects are sharply perceived. Myopia can be corrected by suitable glasses or contact lenses.

Research carried out by a team at the University of Pennsylvania Medical Center in Philadelphia in May 1999 found that the risk of myopia may be increased for infants and toddlers who sleep with a night light turned on. Researchers found that children who had slept in a dark room were far less likely to have developed myopia.

narcotic

Pain-relieving and sleep-inducing drug. The term is usually applied to **heroin**, **morphine**, and other opium derivatives, but may also be used for other drugs which depress brain activity, including anaesthetic agents and hypnotics.

> ❝ Opium is pleasing to the Turks, on account of the agreeable delirium it produces. ❞
>
> **Edmund Burke**, *On the Sublime and Beautiful.*

naturopathy

In **alternative medicine**, facilitating of the natural self-healing processes of the body. Naturopaths are the general practitioners (GPs) of alternative medicine and often refer clients to other specialists, particularly in manipulative therapies, to complement their own work of seeking, through diet, the prescription of natural medicines and supplements, and lifestyle counselling, to restore or augment the vitality of the body and thereby its optimum health.

> ❝ Nature is better than a middling doctor. ❞
>
> **Chinese proverb**.

nerve cell or neurone

Elongated cell, the basic functional unit of the **nervous system** that transmits informa-

Nerve impulses travel quickly – in humans, they may reach speeds of 160 m/525 ft per second.

tion rapidly between different parts of the body. Each nerve cell has a cell body, containing the nucleus, from which trail processes called dendrites, responsible for receiving incoming signals. The unit of information is the nerve impulse, a travelling wave of chemical and electrical changes involving the membrane of the nerve cell. The cell's longest process, the axon, carries impulses away from the cell body.

nervous system

The system of interconnected **nerve cells** composed of the **central nervous system**, comprising the **brain** and **spinal cord** and a peripheral nervous system connecting up with sensory organs, **muscles**, and glands.

neuralgia

Sharp or burning pain originating in a nerve and spreading over its area of distribution. Trigeminal neuralgia, a common form, is a severe pain on one side of the face.

nerve cell *The anatomy and action of a nerve cell. The nerve cell or neurone consists of a cell body with the nucleus and projections called dendrites which pick up messages. An extension of the cell, the axon, connects one cell to the dendrites of the next. When a nerve cell is stimulated, waves of sodium and potassium ions carry an electrical impulse down the axon.*

neurosis

In psychology, a general term referring to emotional disorders, such as **anxiety**, depression, and **phobias**. The main disturbance tends to be one of mood; contact with reality is relatively unaffected, in contrast to **psychosis**.

> ❝ Neurotic means he is not as sensible as I am, and psychotic means he's even worse than my brother-in-law. ❞
>
> **Karl Menninger**, US psychiatrist.

Nightingale, Florence (1820–1910)

English nurse, the founder of nursing as a profession. She took a team of nurses to Scutari (now Üsküdar), Turkey, in 1854 and reduced the Crimean War hospital death rate from 42% to 2%. In 1856 she founded the Nightingale School and Home for Nurses, attached to St Thomas's Hospital, London.

NSAID

Abbreviation for non-steroidal anti-inflammatory drug. Any of a class of drugs used in the treatment of rheumatic or arthritic conditions; they act to reduce pain and swelling in the soft tissues. Bleeding into the digestive tract is a serious side-effect and NSAIDs should not be taken by people with peptic ulcers.

See also: *rheumatoid arthritis.*

nutrition

The science of food and its effects on life, health, and disease. Nutrition involves the study of the basic nutrients required to sustain life, their bioavailability in foods and the effects upon them of cooking and storage. It is also concerned with dietary deficiency diseases.

There are six classes of nutrients: water, **carbohydrates**, **proteins**, **fats**, **vitamins**, and minerals:

- Water is involved in nearly all body processes. A human being will succumb to water deprivation sooner than to starvation.

- Carbohydrates are composed of carbon, hydrogen, and oxygen. The major groups are starches, sugars and cellulose, and related material (or '**roughage**'). The carbohydrates provide energy and serve as efficient sources of glucose, which is needed for brain functioning, utilization of foods, and maintenance of body temperature. Roughage includes the stiff structural materials of vegetables, fruits, and cereals.

- Proteins are made up of smaller units, amino acids. Dietary protein provides the amino acids required for growth and maintenance of body tissues.

- Fats serve as concentrated sources of energy. Saturated fats derive primarily from animal sources; unsaturated fats from vegetable sources such as nuts and seeds.

- Vitamins are essential for normal growth, and are either fat-soluble or water-soluble. Fat-soluble vitamins include A, essential to the maintenance of **mucous membranes**; D, important to the absorption of calcium; E, an anti-oxidant; and K, which aids **blood clotting**. Water-soluble vitamins are the B complex, essential to metabolic reactions, and C, for maintaining **connective tissue**.

- Minerals are vital to normal development. Calcium and iron are required in relatively large amounts; many others are required in trace amounts.

obesity
Condition of being overweight (generally, 20% or more above the desirable weight for one's sex, build, and height). Obesity increases susceptibility to disease, strains the vital organs, and reduces **life expectancy**; it is usually remedied by controlled weight loss, healthy diet, and exercise.

> 6 Obesity is a mental state, a disease brought on by boredom and disappointment. 9
>
> **Cyril Connolly**, *The Unquiet Grave.*

obstetrics
Medical speciality concerned with the management of **pregnancy**, childbirth, and the immediate postnatal period.

occupational therapy
Treatment that aims to assist patients of all ages in overcoming disabilities resulting from physical or psychological illness, accident or old age. The occupational therapist's task is to enable the patient to continue living life to the full and as independently as possible. Occupational therapists work in patients' homes, in hospitals, residential homes, health centres, prisons, and schools. Treatment usually focuses on performing everyday tasks, regaining social skills, building up patients' stamina and self-confidence, and enabling them to return to work if they have jobs. Patients are also advised on how to adapt their homes to meet their specific needs.

oedema

Any abnormal accumulation of fluid in tissues or cavities of the body; waterlogging of the tissues due to excessive loss of **plasma** through the capillary walls. It may be generalized (the condition once known as dropsy) or confined to one area, such as the ankles. Oedema may be mechanical – the result of obstructed veins or heart failure – or it may be due to increased permeability of the capillary walls, as in liver or kidney disease or **malnutrition**. Accumulation of fluid in the abdomen is known as ascites.

oesophagus

Muscular tube by which food travels from the mouth to the stomach. The oesophagus is about 23 cm/9 in long. It extends downwards from the pharynx, immediately behind the windpipe. It is lined with a **mucous membrane** which secretes lubricant fluid to assist the downward movement of food (**peristalsis**).

oestrogen

Any of a group of **hormones** produced by the **ovaries**; the term is also used for various synthetic hormones that mimic their effects. The principal oestrogen is oestradiol. Oestrogens control female sexual development, promote the growth of female second-

US researchers in 1995 observed that oestrogen plays a role in the healing of damaged blood vessels. It has also been found that women recover more quickly from **strokes** if given a low oestrogen dose.

ary sexual characteristics, stimulate egg production, and prepare the lining of the **uterus** for pregnancy. Oestrogens are used therapeutically for some hormone disorders and to inhibit lactation; they also form the basis of oral **contraceptives**.

See also: *hormone replacement therapy, the Pill.*

organ

In biology, part of a living body that has a distinctive function or set of functions. Examples include the liver or brain in animals, or the leaf in plants. An organ is composed of a group of coordinated tissues. A group of organs working together to perform a function is called an organ system, for example, the **digestive system** comprises a number of organs including:

- the **stomach**
- the small intestine
- the colon
- the **pancreas**
- the **liver**.

osteoarthritis

Degenerative form of arthritis which is particularly troublesome when it affects larger, load-bearing joints such as the knee and hip. It appears in later life, especially in joints that have been subject to earlier stress or damage; one or more joints stiffen and may give considerable pain. It is more common in men than women. Treatment of osteoarthritis is primarily conservative. The mainstay is the use of anti-inflammatory drugs (see **NSAID**) and other **analgesics**. **Physiotherapy** is of value and inequalities of leg length due to muscle spasm or bony collapse can be helped with a shoe raise. Surgery may be needed in some cases. Joint replacement surgery is nearly always successful.

See also: *rheumatoid arthritis*.

osteomyelitis

Infection of **bone**, with spread of **pus** along the marrow cavity. Now quite rare, it may follow from a compound fracture (where broken bone protrudes through the skin) or from infectious disease elsewhere in the body. It is more common in children whose bones are not yet fully grown. The symptoms are high fever, severe illness, and pain over the limb. If the infection is at the surface of the bone it may quickly form an **abscess**; if it is deep in the bone marrow it may spread into the circulation and lead to **blood poisoning**. Most cases can be treated with immobilization, **antibiotics**, and surgical drainage.

osteopathy

In **alternative medicine** a system that relies on physical manipulation to treat mechanical stress. It was developed over a century ago by US physician Andrew Taylor Still, who maintained that most ailments can be prevented or cured by techniques of spinal manipulation. Osteopaths are generally consulted to treat problems of the musculo-skeletal structure such as back pain and many doctors refer patients to them. Although in the UK the wider applicability of their skills is not generally recognized, osteopathic doctors in the USA are also fully licensed to practice conventional medicine.

osteoporosis

Disease in which the bone substance becomes porous and brittle and liable to fracture. It is common in older people, affecting more women than men. It may be treated with calcium supplements and drugs known as bisphosphonates. A single **gene** was discovered in 1993 to have a major influence on bone thinning. Osteoporosis may occur in women whose **ovaries** have been removed, unless **hormone-replacement therapy** (HRT) is instituted; it may also occur in Cushing's syndrome and as a side effect of long-term treatment with **corticosteroids**. Early **menopause** in women, childlessness, small body build, lack of exercise, heavy drinking, **smoking**, and **heredity** may be contributory factors.

otitis

Inflammation of the **ear**. *Otitis externa*, occurring in the outer ear canal, is easily treated with **antibiotics**. Inflamed conditions of the middle ear (*otitis media*) or inner ear (*otitis interna*) are more serious, carrying the risk of deafness and infection of the brain. Treatment is with antibiotics or, more rarely, surgery.

A 1999 US survey of childrens' middle-ear problems indicated that the risk is, to a large extent, hereditary.

ovary

In females, the organ that generates the ovum (egg). The ovaries are two whitish rounded bodies about 25 mm/1 in by 35 mm/1.5 in, located in the lower abdomen to either side of the **uterus**. Every month, from **puberty** to the onset of the **menopause**, an ovum is released from the ovary. This is called ovulation, and forms part of the **menstrual cycle**. The ovaries secrete the **hormones** responsible for the secondary sexual characteristics of the female, such as smooth, hairless facial skin, and enlarged breasts. An ovary in a half-grown human **fetus** contains 5 million eggs and so the unborn baby already possesses the female genetic information for the next generation.

palpitation
Condition where a person becomes aware of his or her own heartbeat. This is normal with heightened emotion (fear, excitement) but may also be a symptom of heart disease or **hyperthyroidism**.

pancreas
An accessory gland of the **digestive system** located close to the duodenum. When stimulated by the **hormone** secretin, it releases enzymes into the duodenum that digest starches, **proteins**, and **fats**. It is about 18 cm/7 in long, and lies behind and below the stomach. It contains groups of cells called the islets of Langerhans which secrete the hormones **insulin** and glucagon that regulate the blood sugar level.

panic attack
Sudden, unpredictable episode of overwhelming **anxiety**. It may be accompanied by pronounced physical symptoms, including a racing pulse, overbreathing, dizziness, and sweating.

Paracelsus (1493–1541)
Swiss physician, alchemist, and scientist. He developed the idea that minerals and chemicals might have medical uses (iatrochemistry). He introduced the use of laudanum (which he named) as a

> ❝ Every physician must be rich in knowledge, and not only of that which is written in books; his patients should be his book, they will never mislead him. ❞
>
> **Paracelsus**, *The Book of Tartaric Diseases*, Chapter 13.

pain-killer. His rejection of the ancients and insistence on the value of experimentation make him an important figure in early science.

paracetamol
Analgesic, particularly effective for musculoskeletal pain. It is as effective as **aspirin** in reducing **fever** and less irritating to the stomach but has little anti-inflammatory action. An overdose can cause severe, often irreversible or even fatal, liver and kidney damage.

paralysis
Loss of voluntary movement due to failure of nerve impulses to reach the muscles involved (see **nerve cell**). It may result from almost any disorder of the **nervous system**, including **brain** or **spinal cord** injury, poliomyelitis (**polio**), **stroke**, and progressive conditions such as a **tumour** or **multiple sclerosis**. Paralysis may also involve loss of sensation due to sensory nerve disturbance. Infantile paralysis is an old-fashioned term for polio.

paranoia
Mental disorder marked by delusions of grandeur or persecution. In popular usage, paranoia means baseless or exaggerated fear and suspicion.
See also: *psychosis, schizophrenia.*

paraplegia
Paralysis of the lower limbs, involving loss of both movement and sensation; it is usually due to spinal injury.

Parkinson's disease or parkinsonism
Degenerative disease of the **brain** characterized by a progressive loss of mobility, muscular rigidity, tremor, and speech difficulties. The condition is mainly seen in people over the age of 50. Parkinson's disease destroys a group of cells called the *substantia nigra* ('black substance') in the upper part of the brainstem. These cells are concerned with the production of a neurotransmitter known as dopamine, which is essential to the control of voluntary movement.

The introduction of the drug L-dopa in the 1960s seemed at first the answer to Parkinson's disease. However, it became evident that long-term use brings considerable problems. At best, it postpones the terminal phase of the disease. Brain grafts with dopamine-producing cells were pioneered in the early 1980s and attempts to graft Parkinson's patients with fetal brain tissue have been made. In 1989 a large US study showed that the drug deprenyl may slow the rate at which disability progresses in patients with early Parkinson's disease.

In 1997, the National Human Genome Research Institute at the National Institutes of Health in the USA announced that its scientists had discovered a **gene** that causes Parkinson's disease. According to 1999 research, however, there is strong evidence that environmental factors may also be contributory.

Pasteur, Louis
(1822–1895)

French chemist and microbiologist who discovered that fermentation is caused by micro-organisms, leading to the discovery of the process of pasteurization. He also created a **vaccine** for **rabies**, which led to the foundation of the Pasteur Institute in Paris in 1888. In addition, he developed the germ theory of disease which was probably the most important single medical discovery of all time because it provided both a practical method of combating disease by disinfection and a theoretical foundation for further research.

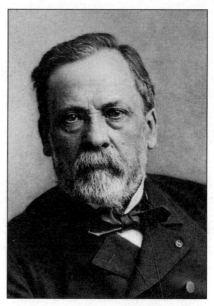

Pasteur *Louis Pasteur developed the theory that disease is caused by germs, probably the most important single medical discovery of all time.*

In 1882, Pasteur began what proved to be his most spectacular research, the prevention of rabies. He demonstrated that the causative **microorganism** (now known to be a

More germs are transmitted when shaking hands than when kissing. Pasteur refused to shake hands with acquaintances for fear of infection.

virus) infects the **nervous system** and then, using the dried tissues of infected animals, he succeeded in obtaining an attenuated form of the virus suitable for the inoculation of human beings. The culmination of this work came on 6 July 1885, when Pasteur used his vaccine to save the life of a young boy who had been bitten by a rabid dog. The success of this experiment led in 1888 to the establishment of the Pasteur Institute, which he headed until his death. He greatly influenced Joseph **Lister** who introduced **antiseptic** surgery.

❝ When meditating over a disease, I never think of finding a remedy for it, but, instead, a means of preventing it. ❞

Pasteur, address to the Fraternal Association of Former Students of the Ecole Centrale des Arts et Manufactures, Paris, 15 May 1884.

pelvis
The lower area of the abdomen featuring the **bones** and **muscles** used to move the legs. The pelvic girdle is a set of bones that allows movement of the legs in relation to the rest of the body and provides sites for the attachment of relevant muscles. The pelvic girdle is formed by the sacrum, the coccyx, and the hip bones; each of the hip bones consists of three originally separate bones, grown together in the adult: the ilium, ischium, and pubis. At the junction of these a socket is formed which takes the ball-end of the **femur**, or thighbone. The pelvic organs for both sexes are the rectum and urinary bladder; for the male, the seminal vesicles and the prostate gland; for the female, the **uterus** and **ovaries**. The female pelvis is broader but shallower and is modified for child-bearing.

Penfield, Wilder Graves (1891–1976)

Canadian neurosurgeon who, while developing surgical options for the treatment of **epilepsy**, located several functional areas of the **cerebral cortex** of the brain. He devised the homunculus, a schematic representation showing the site and relative proportions of the cortical areas specialized for motor and sensory functions.

penicillin

Any of a group of **antibiotic** (bacteria killing) compounds obtained from filtrates of moulds of the genus *Penicillium* (especially *P. notatum*) or produced synthetically. Penicillin was the first antibiotic to be discovered (by Alexander **Fleming**); it kills a broad spectrum of **bacteria**, many of which cause disease in humans. The use of the original type of penicillin is limited by the increasing resistance of pathogens and by allergic reactions (see **allergy**) in patients. Since 1941, numerous other antibiotics of the penicillin family have been discovered.

penis

Male reproductive organ (part of the **genitalia**) containing the urethra (see **urinary system**), the channel through which urine and semen are voided. It transfers sperm to the female reproductive tract to fertilize the ovum. The penis is made erect by vessels that fill with blood.

A 1995 US study showed the average length of an erect human penis to be 12.8 cm/5 in (considerably smaller than is popularly assumed).

periodontal disease

Formerly known as pyorrhoea, disease of the gums and bone supporting the teeth (see **tooth**), caused by the accumulation of plaque and **micro-organisms**; the gums recede and the teeth eventually become loose and may drop out

Australian researchers discovered in 2000 that **aspirin** in low doses might be effective in helping to prevent the disease.

unless treatment is sought. **Bacteria** can eventually erode the bone that supports the teeth so that surgery becomes necessary. Periodontal disease affects an estimated 10% of the world's population. A gel treatment became available early 1997 in Britain and the USA. The gel is applied during surgery and stimulates gum tissue regrowth. About 70% of tissue regrows.

peristalsis
Wavelike contractions, produced by the contraction of smooth **muscle**, that pass along tubular organs such as the **intestines**.
   See also: *digestive system.*

peritoneum
Membrane lining the abdominal cavity and digestive organs. Peritonitis, **inflammation** within the peritoneum, can occur due to infection or other irritation. It is sometimes seen following a burst appendix (see **appendicitis**) and quickly proves fatal if not treated.

persistent vegetative state (PVS)
Condition arising from overwhelming damage to the cerebral cortex. The patient lies unresponsive and, though the eyes may be open, he or she remains unaware of his or her surroundings, makes no purposeful gestures, and never speaks. The vegetative patient may survive for many years in a condition that many observers regard as a living death. However, some patients can regain consciousness, even after as long as five years in a vegetative state.

phenylketonuria (PKU)
Inherited metabolic condition in which the liver of a child cannot control the level of phenylalanine (an amino acid derived from protein foods) in the bloodstream. The condition must be detected promptly (babies are usually tested a few days after birth) and a special diet started in the first few weeks of life if brain damage is to be avoided. Untreated, it causes stunted growth, **epilepsy**, and severe mental disability.

phobia

Excessive irrational fear of an object or situation – for example, **agraphobia** (fear of open spaces and crowded places), acrophobia (fear of heights), and claustrophobia (fear of enclosed places). Behaviour therapy is one form of treatment.

See also: *anxiety.*

physiotherapy

Treatment of injury and disease by physical means such as exercise, heat, manipulation, massage, and electrical stimulation.

PID

Abbreviation for pelvic inflammatory disease, a serious gynaecological condition characterized by lower abdominal pain, malaise, and fever. **Menstruation** may be disrupted; infertility may result. Treatment is with **antibiotics**. The incidence of the disease is twice as high in women using **intrauterine contraceptive devices** (IUDs). PID is potentially life-threatening, and, while mild episodes usually respond to antibiotics, surgery may be necessary in cases of severe or recurrent pelvic infection. The bacterium *Chlamydia trachomatis* has been implicated in a high proportion of cases. The condition is increasingly common.

Piles or haemorrhoids

Distended (**varicose**) **veins** in the area of the anus.

Pill, the

Commonly used term for the **contraceptive** pill based on female **hormones**. The combined pill, which contains synthetic hormones similar to **oestrogen** and **progesterone**, stops the production of eggs (ova) by the **ovaries** and makes the **mucus** produced by the **cervix** hostile to sperm. It is the most reliable form of contraception apart from **sterilization**, being more than 99% effective. The minipill or progesterone-only pill prevents implantation of a fertilized egg into the wall of the **uterus**. The minipill has a slightly higher failure rate, especially if not taken at the same time each day, but has fewer side effects and is considered safer for long-term use. Possible side effects of the Pill include **migraine** or headache and high **blood pressure**. More seriously, oestrogen-containing pills can slightly increase the risk of a clot forming in the blood vessels (**thrombosis**). This risk is increased in women over 35 if they smoke. Controversy surrounds other possible health effects of taking the Pill. The evidence for a link with **cancer** is slight (and the Pill may protect women from some forms of cancer). Once a woman ceases to take the contraceptive pill, there is an increased likelihood of conceiving identical twins.

Pinel, Philippe (1745–1826)
French physician who founded the speciality of **psychiatry** and pioneered the humane treatment of the mentally sick.

pituitary gland
Major **endocrine** gland situated in the centre of the **brain**. It is attached to the hypothalamus by a stalk. The pituitary consists of two lobes. The posterior lobe is an extension of the hypothalamus and is in effect nervous tissue. It stores two hormones synthesized in the hypothalamus: ADH and oxytocin. The anterior lobe secretes six **hormones**, some of which control the activities of other glands (**thyroid**, gonads, and adrenal cortex); others are direct-acting hormones affecting milk secretion and controlling growth.

placebo
(Latin 'I will please'). Any harmless substance, often called a 'sugar pill', that has no active ingredient but may nevertheless bring about improvement in the patient's condition. The use of placebos in medicine is limited to drugs trials, where a placebo may be given alongside the substance being tested to compare effects. The 'placebo effect', first named in 1945, demonstrates the control mind exerts over matter, bringing changes in **blood pressure**, perceived pain, and rates of healing. Recent research points to the release of certain neurotransmitters in the production of the placebo effect.

placenta

Organ that attaches the developing **embryo** or **fetus** to the **uterus**. Composed of maternal and embryonic tissue, it links the blood supply of the embryo to the blood supply of the mother, allowing the exchange of oxygen, nutrients, and waste products. The two blood systems are not in direct contact but are separated by thin membranes, with materials diffusing across from one system to the other. The placenta also produces **hormones** that maintain and regulate pregnancy. It is shed as part of the **afterbirth**. A variety of potentially harmful substances, including drugs and viruses, can pass across the placental membrane.

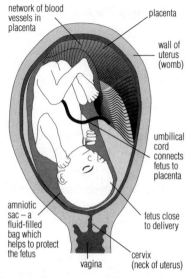

network of blood vessels in placenta

placenta

wall of uterus (womb)

umbilical cord connects fetus to placenta

amniotic sac – a fluid-filled bag which helps to protect the fetus

fetus close to delivery

vagina

cervix (neck of uterus)

placenta *The placenta is a disc-shaped organ about 25 cm/10 in in diameter and 3 cm/ 1 in thick. It is connected to the fetus by the umbilical cord.*

plague

Term applied to any epidemic disease with a high mortality rate, but it usually refers to the bubonic plague. This is a disease transmitted by fleas (carried by the black rat) which infect the sufferer with the bacillus *Yersinia pestis*. An early symptom is swelling of lymph nodes, usually in the armpit and groin; such swellings are

The first description of the plague dates from 40 BC in Libya. The Roman empire was swept by plague during AD 251–260. After the Black Death in the 14th century, plague remained endemic for the next three centuries, the most notorious outbreak being the Great Plague of London in 1665, when about 100,000 of the city's 400,000 inhabitants died.

THE GREAT PLAGUE

In 1666, to help counter the spread of bubonic plague, the British Parliament decreed that all bodies had to be wrapped in a woollen shroud for burial. This decree provided wool-makers with a constant source of business for nearly 150 years.

---

called 'buboes'. It causes virulent **blood poisoning** and the death rate is high. Rarer but more virulent forms of plague are septicaemic and pneumonic. According to a World Health Organization report published in 1996, the incidence of plague is on the increase. In the 1980s and 1990s there were cases in Africa, Latin America, the USA, and southeast Asia. *Y. pestis* persists worldwide in certain wild rodent populations and transmission is mainly by fleas. New plague **vaccines** are under development.

plasma
The liquid component of the **blood**. It is a straw-coloured fluid, largely composed of water (around 90%), in which a number of substances are dissolved. These include a variety of proteins (around 7%) such as fibrinogen (important in **blood clotting**), inorganic mineral salts such as sodium and calcium, waste products such as urea, traces of **hormones**, and **antibodies** to defend against infection.

plastic surgery
Surgical speciality concerned with the repair of congenital defects and the reconstruction of tissues damaged by disease or injury, including burns. If a procedure is undertaken solely for reasons of appearance, for example, the removal of bags under the eyes or a double chin, it is called cosmetic surgery.

pleurisy
Inflammation of the pleura, the thin, secretory membrane that covers the **lungs** and lines the space in which they rest. Pleurisy is nearly always due to bacterial or viral infection (see **bacteria** and **virus**) but

may also be a complication of other diseases. Normally the two lung surfaces move easily on one another, lubricated by small quantities of fluid. When the pleura is inflamed, the surfaces may dry up or stick together, making breathing difficult and painful. Alternatively, a large volume of fluid may collect in the pleural cavity, the space between the two surfaces, and **pus** may accumulate.

pneumonia
Inflammation of the **lungs**, generally due to bacterial or viral infection (see **bacteria** and **virus**). It is characterized by a buildup of fluid in the alveoli, the clustered air sacs (at the ends of the air passages) where oxygen exchange takes place. Symptoms include fever and pain in the chest. With widespread availability of **antibiotics**, infectious pneumonia is much less common than it was. However, it remains a dire threat to patients whose immune systems are suppressed (including **transplant** recipients and **AIDS** and **cancer** victims) and to those who are critically ill or injured. Pneumocystis pneumonia is a leading cause of death in AIDS.

pneumothorax
The presence of air in the pleural cavity, between a **lung** and the chest wall. Prevented from expanding normally, the lung is liable to collapse. It may be due to a penetrating injury of the lung or to lung disease, or it may occur without apparent cause (spontaneous pneumothorax) in an otherwise healthy person.

poison or toxin
Any chemical substance that, when introduced into or applied to the body, is capable of injuring health or destroying life. The **liver** removes some poisons from the blood. The majority of poisons may be divided into:

- corrosives, such as sulphuric, nitric, and hydrochloric acids;
- irritants, including arsenic and copper sulphate;
- **narcotics** such as opium and carbon monoxide;
- and narcotico-irritants from any substances of plant origin including carbolic acid and tobacco.

In the UK, the National Poisons Information Service, which was founded 1963, provides eight regional centres in major city hospitals, where data on cases of poisoning is collected. Poisoning incidents (mostly self-poisonings) are a major cause of admission to acute medical wards.

polio
(Abbreviation for poliomyelitis) Viral infection (see **virus**) of the **central nervous system** affecting nerves that activate muscles. The disease used to be known as infantile **paralysis** since children were most often affected. Two kinds of **vaccine** are available, one injected and one given by mouth.
- The Americas were declared polio-free in 1994.
- In 1988 when the World Health Organization (WHO) launched its eradication programme there were 35,000 cases worldwide; within a decade 82% of the world's children had been vaccinated and only 3,200 cases were known (a third of these in India).
- The target date for the final eradication of polio is the year 2050.

> ❝ The people – could you patent the sun? ❞
>
> **Jonas E Salk**, on being asked who owned the patent on his polio vaccine, quote in *Famous Men of Science*.

polyp or polypus
Small 'stalked' benign **tumour**, usually found on **mucous membrane** of the nose or bowels. Intestinal polyps are usually removed since some have been found to be precursors of **cancer**.

Postmortem or autopsy
Dissection of a dead body to determine the cause of death.

pre-eclampsia
(Or toxaemia of **pregnancy**) Potentially serious condition developing in the third trimester and marked by high **blood pressure** and fluid

retention (**oedema**). Arising from unknown causes, it disappears when pregnancy is over. It may progress to the life-threatening condition known as eclampsia if untreated.

pregnancy

The process during which a developing **embryo** grows within the woman's womb. It begins at conception (see **fertilization**) and ends at birth. The normal length of pregnancy is 40 weeks, around nine months.

Menstruation (see **menstrual cycle**) usually stops on conception. About one in five

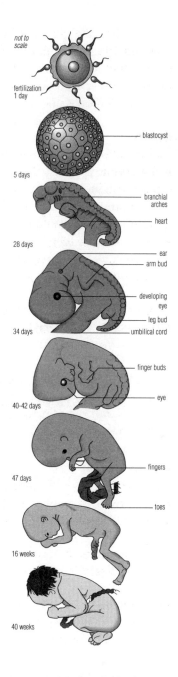

not to scale

fertilization
1 day

blastocyst

5 days

branchial arches

heart

28 days

ear

arm bud

developing eye

leg bud

umbilical cord

34 days

finger buds

eye

40-42 days

fingers

47 days

toes

16 weeks

40 weeks

pregnancy *The development of a human embryo. Division of the fertilized egg, or ovum, begins within hours of conception. Within a week a ball of cells –a blastocyst – has developed. After the third week, the embryo has changed from a mass of cells into a recognizable shape. At four weeks, the embryo is 3 mm/0.1 in long, with a large bulge for the heart and small pits for the ears. At six weeks, the embryo is 1.5 cm/0.6 in with a pulsating heart and ear flaps. At the eighth week, the embryo is 2.5 cm/ 1 in long and recognizably human, with eyelids, small fingers, and toes. From the end of the second month, the embryo is almost fully formed and further development is mainly by growth. After this stage, the embryo is termed a fetus.*

pregnancies fails, but most do so very early on so the woman may notice only that her period (loss of blood) is late. After the second month, the breasts become tender and the areolae round the nipples become darker. Enlargement of the **uterus** can be felt at about the end of the third month and after this the abdomen enlarges progressively. **Fetal** movement can be felt at about 18 weeks; a **heartbeat** may be heard during the sixth month.

prematurity

The condition of an infant born before the full term. In obstetrics, an infant born before 37 weeks' gestation (see **pregnancy**) is described as premature. Premature babies are often at risk. They lose heat quickly because they lack an insulating layer of fat beneath the skin; there may also be breathing difficulties. In hospitals with advanced technology, specialized neonatal units can save some babies born as early as 23 weeks.

premenstrual tension

(PMT or premenstrual syndrome) Medical condition caused by **hormone** changes and comprising a number of physical and emotional features that occur cyclically before **menstruation** and disappear with its onset. Symptoms include mood changes, breast tenderness, a feeling of bloatedness, and headache.

Controversially, in 1993 the American Psychiatric Association decided to rename premenstrual syndrome and to categorize sufferers as being mentally ill. The Association estimates that 5% of US women suffer from the condition, now designated premenstrual dysphoric disorder (PMDD), recognized as a condition requiring medical treatment.

pressure sore or decubitus ulcer

Ulceration caused by continuous pressure on part of the body, particularly on a bony prominence such as the sacrum or the heel. It is aggravated by reduced blood supply to the area and local **gangrene** may develop. It is notoriously hard to treat. Pressure sores may occur at any age but are particularly common in the frail elderly confined to bed for any length of time. They may develop within an hour of a vulnerable patient being left on a hard, unyielding hospital trolley. Nurses are concerned to prevent pressure sores by frequent turning of patients who are confined to bed. Pressure sores are commonly known as bedsores.

progesterone
Steroid **hormone** that regulates the **menstrual cycle** and **pregnancy**. Progesterone is secreted by the corpus luteum (the ruptured Graafian follicle of a discharged ovum).

prophylaxis
Any measure taken to prevent disease, including exercise and vaccination (see **vaccine**). Prophylactic (preventive) medicine is an aspect of public-health provision that is receiving increasing attention.

prostate gland
Gland surrounding and opening into the urethra at the base of the bladder in males. The prostate gland produces an alkaline fluid that is released during ejaculation; this fluid activates **sperm**, and prevents their clumping together. Older men may develop benign prostatic hyperplasia (BPH), a painful condition in which the prostate becomes enlarged and restricts urine flow. This can cause further problems of the bladder and kidneys. The condition is treated surgically.

protein
Complex, biologically important substance composed of amino acids joined by peptide bonds. Proteins are essential to all living organisms. As enzymes they regulate all aspects of **metabolism**. Structural proteins such as keratin and collagen make up the skin, bones, tendons, and ligaments; muscle proteins produce movement; **haemoglobin** transports oxygen; and membrane proteins regulate the movement of substances into and out of cells. Protein is an

essential part of the diet (see **nutrition**), and is found in greatest quantity in soy beans and other grain legumes, meat, eggs, and cheese.

pruritus
Itching, usually caused by irritation of the skin.

psoriasis
Chronic, recurring skin disease characterized by raised, red, scaly patches on the scalp, elbows, knees, and elsewhere. Tar preparations, steroid creams, and ultraviolet light are used to treat the condition and sometimes it disappears spontaneously. Psoriasis may be accompanied by a form of arthritis (inflammation of the joints). In 1999 a **vaccine** (PVAC) successfully completed its clinical trials proving to be effective in half the cases treated. PVAC is the first vaccine to eradicate a disease already prevalent in the body. It works by disrupting the body's T lymphocytes, part of the immune response, that are attacking the skin cells. It is a common disease, sometimes running in families, and affects 100 million people worldwide. It affects about 2% of the UK population.

psychiatry
Branch of medicine dealing with the diagnosis and treatment of mental disorder, normally divided into the areas of neurotic conditions (neurosis), including **anxiety**, depression, and **hysteria**; and **psychotic** disorders, such as **schizophrenia**. Psychiatric treatment consists of drugs, analysis, or electroconvulsive therapy. In practice there is considerable overlap between psychiatry and clinical psychology, the fundamental difference being that psychiatrists are trained medical doctors (holding an MD degree) and may therefore

6 Psychiatry's chief contribution to philosophy is the discovery that the toilet is the seat of the soul. 9

Alexander Chase, US journalist, *Perspectives*.

prescribe drugs, whereas psychologists may hold a PhD but do not need a medical qualification to practise.

See also: *psychoanalysis.*

psychoanalysis

Theory and treatment method for neuroses (see **neurosis**), developed by Austrian psychiatrist Sigmund Freud in the 1890s. Psychoanalysis asserts that the impact of early childhood sexuality and experiences, stored in the unconscious, can lead to the development of adult emotional problems. The main treatment method involves the free association of ideas, and their interpretation by patient and analyst. Psychoanalytic treatment aims to free the patient from specific symptoms and from irrational inhibitions and anxieties. In the early 1900s a group of psychoanalysts gathered around Freud. Some of these later broke away and formed their own schools, notably Alfred Adler (also Austrian) in 1911 and Carl Jung in Switzerland in 1913. The significance of early infantile experience has been further elaborated in the field of child analysis, particularly in the work of Melanie Klein in Austria, and her students, who pay particular attention to the development of the infant in the first six to eight months of life.

> ❛ Psychoanalysis is spending 40 dollars an hour to squeal on your mother. ❜
>
> **Mike Connolly**, quoted in *Bartlett's Unfamiliar Quotations.*

psychosis or psychotic disorder

General term for a serious mental disorder where the individual commonly loses contact with reality and may experience **hallucinations** (seeing or hearing things that do not exist) or delusions (fixed false beliefs). For example, in a paranoid psychosis (see **paranoia**) an individual may believe that others are plotting against him or her. A major type of psychosis is **schizophrenia**.

psychosurgery
Operation to relieve severe mental illness.

puberty
Stage in human development when the individual becomes sexually mature. It may occur from the age of ten upwards. The sexual organs take on their adult form and pubic hair grows. In girls, **menstruation** begins and the breasts develop; in boys, the voice breaks and becomes deeper and facial hair develops.

pus
Yellowish fluid that forms in the body as a result of bacterial infection; it includes **white blood cells** (leucocytes), living and dead **bacteria**, dead tissue, and serum. An enclosed collection of pus is called an **abscess**.

quarantine
Any period for which people, animals, plants, or vessels may be detained in isolation to prevent the spread of contagious disease.

quinine
Drug extracted from the bark of the cinchona tree, used against the parastic disease **malaria**. Peruvian Indians taught French missionaries how to use the bark in 1630 but quinine was not isolated until 1820. It is a bitter alkaloid. Other antimalarial drugs have since been developed with fewer side effects, but quinine derivatives are still valuable in the treatment of unusually resistant strains of the disease.

quinsy or peritonsillar abscess
Abscess in the soft palate near one of the **tonsils**. It may occur in tonsillitis.

rabies or hydrophobia

Viral disease (see **virus**) of the **central nervous system** that can afflict all warm-blooded creatures. It is almost invariably fatal once symptoms have developed. Its transmission to humans is generally by a bite from an infected animal. Rabies continues to kill hundreds of thousands of people every year; almost all these deaths occur in Asia, Africa, and South America. After an incubation period, which may vary from ten days to more than a year, symptoms of fever, muscle spasm, and delirium develop. As the disease progresses the mere sight of water is enough to provoke **convulsions** and **paralysis**. Death is usual within four or five days from the onset of symptoms. Injections of rabies **vaccine** and antiserum may save those bitten by a rabid animal from developing the disease. Louis **Pasteur** was the first to produce an anti-rabies vaccine.

Rabies has been virtually eradicated in Western Europe and no one has died of the disease in the European Union (EU) since 1973. In Britain, no human rabies has been transmitted since 1902. Britain and Ireland are the only countries in the EU to quarantine incoming pets (for a six-month period). However, since 1999, animals from the EU, and rabies-free islands such as Australia and New Zeland, have been allowed into the UK without a period of quarantine as long as a full course of required vaccination has been administered to the animal.

radiation sickness

Sickness resulting from exposure to radiation, including X-rays, gamma rays, neutrons, and other nuclear radiation, as from weapons and fallout. Such radiation ionizes atoms in the body and causes nausea, vomiting, diarrhoea, and other symptoms. The body cells themselves may be damaged even by very small doses, causing **leukaemia** and other **cancers**.

radioisotope scanning

Use of radioactive materials (radioisotopes or radionucleides) to pinpoint disease. It reveals the size and shape of the target organ and whether any part of it is failing to take up radioactive material, usually an indication of disease. The speciality known as nuclear medicine makes use of the affinity of different chemical elements for certain parts of the body. Iodine, for instance, always makes its way to the **thyroid** gland. After being made radioactive, these materials can be given by mouth or injected and then traced on scanners working on the Geiger-counter principle. The diagnostic record gained from radioisotope scanning is known as a scintigram.

radiology

Medical speciality concerned with the use of radiation, including X-rays, and radioactive materials in the diagnosis and treatment of injury and disease.

radiotherapy

Treatment of disease by radiation from X-ray machines or radioactive sources. Radiation, which reduces the activity of dividing cells, is of special value for its effect on malignant tissues (see **cancer**), certain nonmalignant **tumours**, and some diseases of the skin. Generally speaking, the rays of the diagnostic X-ray machine are not penetrating enough to be efficient in treatment, so for this purpose more powerful machines are required, operating from 10,000 to over 30 million volts. The lower-voltage machines are similar to conventional X-ray machines; the higher-voltage ones may be of special design; for example, linear accelerators and betatrons. Modern radiotherapy is associated with fewer side effects than formerly but radiotherapy to the head can cause temporary hair loss, and, if the treatment involves the gut, diarrhoea and vomiting may occur. Much radiation now given uses synthesized radioisotopes. Radioactive cobalt is the most useful since it produces gamma rays, which are highly penetrating, and it is used instead of very high-energy X-rays.

Similarly, certain radioactive substances may be administered to patients; for example, radioactive iodine for thyroid disease.

Radium, formerly widely used for radiotherapy, has now been supplanted by artificially produced substances.

Raynaud's disease

Chronic condition in which the blood supply to the extremities is reduced by periodic spasm of the blood vessels on exposure to cold. It is most often seen in young women. Attacks are usually brought on by cold-weather conditions or by emotional factors. Typically, the hands and/or feet take on a corpselike pallor, changing to blue as the circulation begins to return when initial numbness is replaced by a tingling or burning sensation. Drugs may be necessary to control the condition, which in exceptional cases can give rise to ulceration or **gangrene**.

recovery position

Body position used to safeguard an unconscious patient until medical help arrives. The person is placed lying on one side with the uppermost shoulder tilted towards the ground and the knees half drawn up so that any regurgitated matter is able to drain freely from the mouth.

red blood cell or erythrocyte

The most common type of blood cell, responsible for transporting oxygen around the body. It contains **haemoglobin**, which combines with oxygen from the **lungs** to form oxyhaemoglobin. When transported to the tissues, these cells are able to release the oxygen because the oxyhaemoglobin splits into its original constituents. Erythrocytes are disc-shaped with a depression in the centre and no nucleus; they are manufactured in the bone marrow and last for only four months before being destroyed in the **liver** and **spleen**.

reflexology

In **alternative medicine**, manipulation and massage of the feet to ascertain and treat disease or dysfunction elsewhere in the body. Correspondence between reflex points on the feet and remote organic and physical functions were discovered early in the 20th century by US physician William Fitzgerald, who also found that pressure and massage applied to these reflex points beneficially affect the related organ or function.

relaxation therapy

Development of regular and conscious control of physiological processes and their related emotional and mental states, and of muscular tensions in the body, as a way of relieving stress, and its symptoms. Meditation, hypnotherapy, autogenics, and biofeedback are techniques commonly employed.

repetitive strain injury (RSI)

Inflammation of **tendon** sheaths, mainly in the hands and wrists, which may be disabling. It is found predominantly in factory workers involved in constant repetitive movements and in those who work at computer keyboards. The symptoms include aching **muscles**, weak wrists, tingling fingers and, in severe cases, pain and **paralysis**. Some victims have successfully sued their employers and have been awarded financial compensation.

In 1999 it was established that RSI affected more than a million people annually in Britain and the USA.

resuscitation

Steps taken to revive anyone on the brink of death. The most successful technique for life-threatening emergencies, such as electrocution, near-drowning, or **heart attack**, is mouth-to-mouth resuscitation. Medical and paramedical staff are trained in cardiopulmonary resuscitation (CPR): the use of specialized equipment and techniques to attempt to restart the breathing and/or **heartbeat** and stabilize the patient long enough for more definitive treatment. CPR has a success rate of less than 30%.

Reye's syndrome

Rare disorder of the **metabolism** causing fatty infiltration of the **liver** and **encephalitis**. It occurs mainly in children and has been linked with aspirin therapy, although its cause is still uncertain. The mortality rate is 50%.

rhesus factor

Group of antigens on the surface of **red blood cells** which characterize the rhesus blood group system. Most individuals possess the main rhesus factor (Rh+), but those without this factor (Rh–) produce **antibodies** if they come into contact with it. The name comes from rhesus monkeys, in whose blood rhesus factors were first found. If an Rh– mother carries an Rh+ fetus, she may produce antibodies if fetal blood crosses the **placenta**. This is not normally a problem with the first infant because antibodies are only produced slowly. However, the antibodies continue to build up after birth and a second Rh+ baby may be attacked by antibodies passing from mother to **fetus**, causing the child to develop **anaemia**, heart failure, or brain damage. In such cases, the blood of the infant has to be exchanged for Rh– blood; a badly affected fetus may be treated in the womb. The problem can be circumvented by giving the mother anti-Rh globulin just after the first pregnancy, preventing the formation of antibodies. Rhesus disease of the newborn is now quite rare.

rheumatic fever or acute rheumatism

Acute or chronic illness characterized by fever and painful swelling of joints. Some victims also experience involuntary movements of the limbs and head, a form of the disease of the **central nervous system**, chorea. It is now rare in the developed world. Rheumatic fever, which strikes mainly children and young adults, is always preceded by a streptococcal infection such as scarlet fever or a severe sore throat, usually occurring a couple of weeks beforehand. It is treated with bed rest, **antibiotics**, and painkillers. The most important complication of rheumatic fever is damage to the heart and its valves, producing rheumatic heart disease many years later.

rheumatism

Nontechnical term for a variety of ailments associated with **inflammation** and stiffness of the joints and **muscles**. Acute rheumatism is better known as rheumatic fever.

> 6 We don't believe in rheumatism and true love until after the first attack. 9
> **Maria Ebner von Eschenbach**, Austrian writer, attributed remark.

rheumatoid arthritis

Inflammation of the joints. A chronic progressive disease, it begins with pain and stiffness in the small joints of the hands and feet and spreads to involve other joints, often with severe disability and disfigurement. There may also be damage to the eyes, **nervous system,** and other organs. In children rheumatoid arthritis is known as 'Still's disease'. Rheumatoid arthritis most often develops between the ages of 30 and 40 and is three times more common in women than men. It is an autoimmune disease. Remissions alternating with exacerbations occur. About 50% of cases remain stationary for many years, while other cases become progressively worse. Treatment consists of rest and in preventing, by splinting and other means, the development of deformities. **Physiotherapy** encourages active and passive movements and generally maintains muscle tone. Gold injections have proved helpful in some cases. Simple **aspirin** or codeine tablets are valuable in relieving pain. Anti-inflammatory drugs (see **NSAIDs**) also may bring considerable relief from pain. Other compounds that are used with some success include penicillamine and **cytotoxic** drugs.

The use of total joint replacements in the hand, hip, and knee in particular, has helped many people to regain some degree of pain-free mobility.

rhinitis

Inflammation of the **mucous membrane** of the nose. It may be caused by **virus** infection (for example the **common cold**) or by some allergen (see allergy), as in **hay fever**.

RNA (ribonucleic acid)

Nucleic acid involved in the process of translating the genetic material **DNA** into **proteins**. It is usually single-stranded, unlike the double-stranded DNA, and consists of a large number of nucleotides strung together, each of which comprises the sugar ribose, a phosphate group, and one of four bases (uracil, cytosine, adenine, or guanine). RNA is copied from DNA by the formation of base pairs, with uracil taking the place of thymine.

Although RNA is normally associated only with the process of protein synthesis, it makes up the hereditary material itself in some **viruses**, such as retroviruses.

Röntgen, Wilhelm Konrad (1845–1923)

German physicist who discovered X-rays in 1895. While investigating the passage of electricity through gases, he noticed the fluorescence of a barium platinocyanide screen. This radiation passed through some substances opaque to light and affected photographic plates. Developments from this discovery revolutionized medical diagnosis. He won the Nobel Prize for Physics in 1901.

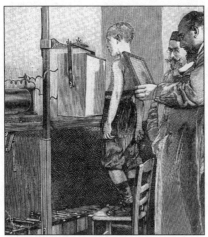

Röntgen *Wilhelm Röntgen making an early diagnosis of pulmonary tuberculosis using his new X-ray technology.*

❝ X-RAYS: Their moral is this – that a right way of looking at things will see through almost anything. ❞

Samuel Butler, *Note-Books,* Vol V.

Today, the unit of radiation exposure is called the roentgen, or röntgen (symbol R). Röntgen refused to make any financial gain out of his findings, believing that the products of scientific research should be made freely available to all.

roughage

Alternative term for dietary fibre: material of plant origin that cannot be digested by enzymes normally present in the human gut.
  See also: *nutrition.*

rubella

Technical term for **German measles**.

Sabin, Albert Bruce (1906–1903)

Russian-born US virologist who developed a live virus oral **vaccine** against poliomyelitis (see **polio**). Introduced in 1957, it replaced the inactivated virus vaccine pioneered five years previously by Jonas Salk.

salmonella

Any of a very varied group of **bacteria**, genus *Salmonella*, that colonize the intestines of humans and some animals. Some strains cause typhoid and paratyphoid fevers, while others cause salmonella food poisoning, which is characterized by stomach pains, vomiting, **diarrhoea**, and headache. It can be fatal in elderly people, but others usually recover in a few days without antibiotics. Most cases are caused by contaminated animal products, especially poultry meat. Human carriers of the disease may be well themselves but pass the bacteria on to others through unhygienic preparation of food. Domestic pets can also carry the bacteria while appearing healthy.

scanning

The noninvasive examination of body organs to detect abnormalities of structure or function. Detectable waves – for example, ultrasound, gamma, or X-rays – are passed through the part to be scanned. Their absorption pattern is recorded, analysed by computer and displayed pictorially on a screen. Diagnostic scanning can also be caried out using **magnetic resonance imaging** (MRI) or **radiosotope scanning**.

scapula or shoulder blade

Large, flat, triangular bone which lies over the second to seventh ribs on the back, forming part of the pectoral girdle and assisting in the articulation of the arm with the chest region. Its flattened shape allows a large region for the attachment of **muscles**.

schizophrenia

Mental disorder, a **psychosis** of unknown origin, which can lead to profound changes in personality, behaviour, and perception, including delusions and **hallucinations**. It is more common in males and the early-onset form is more severe than when the illness develops in later life. Modern treatment approaches include drugs, family therapy, stress reduction, and rehabilitation.

Schizophrenia implies a severe divorce from reality in the patient's thinking. Although the causes are poorly understood, it is now recognized as an organic disease, associated with structural anomalies in the **brain**. There is some evidence that early trauma, either in the womb or during delivery, may play a part in causation. There is also a genetic contribution.

- Paranoid schizophrenia, characterized by feelings of persecution, is 50% more common in developed countries.
- Catatonic schizophrenia, characterized by total immobility, is six times more frequent in developing countries.
- Hebephrenic schizophrenia, characterized by disorganized behaviour and speech and emotional bluntness, is four times more prevalent in developed countries overall but is rare in the USA.

The prevalence of schizophrenia in Europe is about two to five cases per 1,000 of the population.

See also: *paranioa*.

---

6 Schizophrenia cannot be understood without understanding despair. 9

R D Laing, British psychiatrist, *The Divided Self.*

---

sciatica

Persistent pain in the back and down the outside of one leg, along the sciatic nerve and its branches. Causes of sciatica include **inflammation** of the nerve or pressure of a displaced disc on a nerve root leading out of the lower spine.

seasonal affective disorder (SAD)
Form of depression that occurs in winter and is relieved by the coming of spring. Its incidence decreases closer to the Equator. One type of SAD is associated with increased sleeping and appetite. Symptoms in some sufferers can be alleviated by the use of a 'light box' which exposes the user to artificial sunlight.

It has been suggested that SAD may be caused by changes in the secretion of melatonin, a **hormone** produced by the pineal body in the brain. Melatonin secretion is inhibited by bright daylight.

sedative
Any drug that has a calming effect, reducing **anxiety** and tension. Sedatives will induce sleep in larger doses. Examples are barbiturates, **narcotics**, and benzodiazepines.

semen
Fluid containing **sperm** from the **testes** and secretions from various sex glands (such as the **prostate gland**) that is ejaculated by the male animal during copulation. The secretions serve to nourish and activate the sperm cells and prevent them clumping together.

senile dementia
Dementia associated with old age, often caused by **Alzheimer's disease.**

sepsis
General term for infectious change in the body caused by **bacteria** or their **toxins**.

septicaemia
General term for any form of **blood poisoning**.

serotonin

A chemical widely distributed in the body tissues – in the blood platelets, the wall of the intestine, and the **central nervous system**. It is believed to be implicated in the inflammatory process and, in the nervous system, it acts as a neurotransmitter, controlling sleep. Serotonin is synthesized from the amino acid tryptophan.

severe combined immune deficiency (SCID)

Rare condition caused by a **gene** malfunction in which a baby is born unable to produce the enzyme ADA. Without ADA the T cells involved in fighting infection are poisoned; untreated infants usually die before the age of two. The child must be kept within a germ-free bubble, a transparent plastic tent, until a matched donor can provide a bone-marrow transplant (bone marrow is the source of disease-fighting cells in the body).

There have been promising results from experimental gene therapy for this condition, pioneered in the USA; in 1993 doctors inserted the ADA gene into stem cells from the umbilical cords of three babies born with SCID and reintroduced them. The gene was still present in blood cells in 1995, though only in 1% of T cells. The percentage will need to increase to a minimum of 10% for additional drug treatment to become possibly unnecessary.

sex chromosome

Chromosome that differs between the sexes and that serves to determine the sex of the individual. Females have two X chromosomes and males have an X and a Y chromosome.

sexually transmitted disease (STD)

Any disease transmitted by sexual contact, involving transfer of body fluids. STDs include not only the traditional venereal diseases but also a growing list of conditions, such as **AIDS** and scabies, which are known to be spread primarily by sexual contact. Other diseases that are transmitted sexually include viral **hepatitis**.

The World Health Organization (WHO) estimate that there are 356,000 new cases of STDs daily worldwide (1995).

shiatsu
In **alternative medicine**, Japanese method of massage derived from **acupuncture** and sometimes referred to as '**acupressure**', which treats organic or physiological dysfunctions by applying finger or palm pressure to parts of the body remote from the affected part.

shingles
Common name for **herpes** zoster, a disease characterized by infection of sensory nerves, with pain and eruption of **blisters** along the course of the affected nerves.

shock
Term used to describe circulatory failure marked by a sudden fall in **blood pressure** and resulting in pallor, sweating, fast (but weak) pulse, and sometimes complete collapse. Causes include disease, injury, and psychological trauma. In shock, the blood pressure falls below that necessary to supply the tissues of the body, especially the brain. Treatment depends on the cause. Rest is needed, and, in the case of severe blood loss, restoration of the normal circulating volume.

short-sightedness or myopia
Defect of the eye in which a person can see clearly only those objects that are close up. It is caused by either the eyeball being too long or by the cornea and lens system of the eye being too powerful, both of which cause the images of distant objects to be formed in front of the retina. Short-sightedness can be corrected by wearing spectacles fitted with diverging lenses or by wearing diverging (concave meniscus) contact lenses.

sick building syndrome
Malaise diagnosed in the early 1980s among office workers and thought to be caused by chemical pollutants such as formaldehyde (from furniture and insulating materials), benzene (from paint), and the solvent trichloroethene, concentrated in air-conditioned buildings. Symptoms include headache, sore throat, tiredness, colds, and

influenza. Studies have found that it can cause a 40% drop in productivity and a 30% rise in absenteeism.

sickle-cell disease or sickle-cell anaemia

Hereditary chronic blood disorder common among people of black African descent; also found in the eastern Mediterranean, parts of the Persian Gulf, and in northeastern India. It is characterized by distortion and fragility of the **red blood cells**, which are lost too rapidly from the circulation.

The disease is caused by a recessive allele (**genes** responsible for alternative characteristics). People born with two copies of the recessive allele suffer debilitating **anaemia**; those with only a single copy paired with the normal allele suffer only mild anaemia. About 100,000 babies are born worldwide with the disorder each year.

> People with the milder form of the disease have a degree of protection against **malaria** because fewer normal red blood cells are available to the parasites for infection.

side effect

An effect, usually undesirable, that accompanies the therapeutic effect for which a particular drug has been administered. Side effects range from mild to severe and include drowsiness, induced by many **antibiotics** and **antihistamine** tablets, and, in the case of some tranquillizers, partial **paralysis** and blurred vision.

sinusitis

Painful **inflammation** of one of the sinuses, or air spaces, that surround nasal passages. Most cases clear with **antibiotics** and nasal decongestants but some require surgical drainage. Sinusitis most frequently involves the maxillary sinuses within the cheek bones, producing pain around the eyes, toothache, and a nasal discharge.

skeleton

The rigid or semirigid framework that supports and gives form to the body, protects the internal organs, and provides anchorage points for

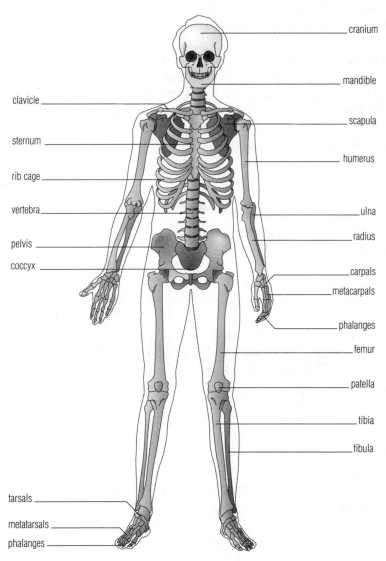

cranium

mandible

clavicle

scapula

sternum

humerus

rib cage

vertebra

ulna

pelvis

radius

coccyx

carpals

metacarpals

phalanges

femur

patella

tibia

fibula

tarsals

metatarsals

phalanges

skeleton *The human skeleton is made up of 206 bones and provides a strong but flexible supportive framework for the body.*

the **muscles**. The human skeleton is composed of 206 bones, with the vertebral column (**spine**) forming the central supporting structure.

skin

The covering of the body. The outer layer (epidermis) is dead and its cells are constantly being rubbed away and replaced from below; it helps to protect the body from infection and to prevent dehydration. The lower layer (dermis), con-

A US biotechnology company applied for permission to the US Food and Drug Administration in 1995 to begin mass-production of human skin. Sheets of skin are grown on biodegradable polymer scaffolds seeded by fibroblast cells taken from the foreskins of circumcised infants. This and another artificial skin product, a matrix constructed from bovine collagen and shark cartilage, was approved in 1997 by the US Food and Drug Administration.

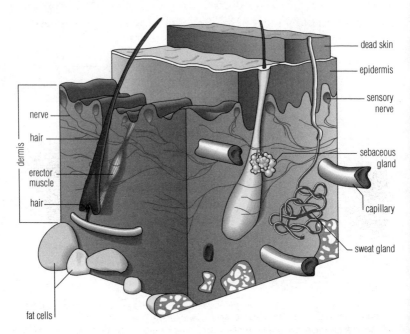

skin *The skin of an adult man covers about 1.9 sq m/20 sq ft; a woman's skin covers about 1.6 sq m/17 sq ft. During our lifetime, we shed about 18 kg/40 lb of skin.*

taining blood vessels, nerves, hair roots, and sweat and sebaceous glands, is supported by a network of fibrous and elastic cells. The medical speciality concerned with skin diseases is called dermatology. Skin grafting is the repair of injured skin by placing pieces of skin, taken from elsewhere on the body, over the injured area.

skull

The collection of flat and irregularly shaped bones (or cartilage) that enclose the **brain** and the organs of sight, hearing, and smell and provide support for the jaws. The skull consists of 22 bones joined by fibrous immobile joints called sutures. The floor of the skull is pierced by a large hole (*foramen magnum*) for the **spinal cord** and a number of smaller apertures through which other nerves and blood vessels pass. The skull comprises the cranium (brain case) and the bones of the face, which include the upper jaw, enclosing the sinuses, and form the framework for the nose, eyes, and the roof of the mouth. The lower jaw is hinged to the middle of the skull at its lower edge. The opening to

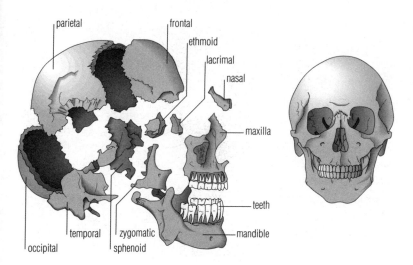

skull *The skull is a protective box for the brain, eyes, and hearing organs. It is also a framework for the teeth and flesh of the face. The cranium has eight bones: occipital, two temporal, two parietal, frontal, sphenoid, and ethmoid. The face has 14 bones, the main ones being two maxillae, two nasal, two zygoma, two lacrimal, and the mandible.*

the middle ear is located near the jaw hinge. The plate at the back of the head is jointed at its lower edge with the upper section of the spine. Inside, the skull has various shallow cavities into which fit different parts of the brain.

slipped disc
(Or prolapsed intervertebral disc.) Protrusion of the soft inner substance of an intervertebral disc through the outer covering, causing pressure on nerve roots. It is caused by heavy or awkward lifting or sudden twisting of the spine or bending. Symptoms are severe pain, with **sciatica**, and immobility. There is a range of treatments available, including bed rest, traction, or **osteopathy** and **analgesics**.

smallpox
Acute, highly contagious viral disease marked by aches, fever, vomiting, and skin eruptions which leave pitted scars. Smallpox was common in Europe until the development of vaccination (see **vaccine**) by Edward **Jenner,** about 1800, and remained so in Asia, where a virulent form of the disease (*variola major*) was fatal to 30% of victims until the World Health Organization (WHO) campaign from 1967, which resulted in its virtual disappearance by 1980. The campaign was estimated to have cost $300 million/£200 million and was the organization's biggest health success to date.

• In June 1996 the WHO agreed to wipe out all traces of the smallpox **virus** by the end of the century by destroying the 400 remaining samples of *variola* locked in special freezers at various research institutes. This agreement followed fears that if the virus escaped it could be lethal, as populations are no longer considered to have **immunity**.

• In 1999 the WHO postponed the date for final destruction of the last remaining smallpox samples, promising to set a new deadline by 2002. Fears of the existence of unofficial stocks of smallpox and the possible use of the virus by bioterrorists were behind the postponement.

smoking
Inhaling the fumes from burning substances, generally tobacco in the

form of cigarettes. The practice is habit-forming and is dangerous to health, since carbon monoxide and other toxic materials result from the

In China there were 300 million smokers in 1999.

combustion process. A direct link between lung **cancer** and tobacco smoking was established in 1950; the habit is also linked to respiratory and coronary **heart** diseases. In the West, smoking is now forbidden in many public places because even passive smoking – breathing in fumes from other people's cigarettes – can be harmful. Manufacturers have attempted to filter out harmful substances such as tar and nicotine, and to use milder tobaccos, and governments have carried out extensive antismoking advertising campaigns. In the UK and the USA all cigarette packaging must carry a government health warning and television advertising of cigarettes is forbidden, although other forms of advertising are widespread. Scientific studies have revealed considerable evidence of nicotine's addictive properties, showing that it acts on the brain in the same way as addictive drugs, releasing the 'feel-good' chemical dopamine. The US Food and Drug Administration officially accepted that nicotine is an addictive drug in 1996. In developing countries, China and southeast Asia, where health education has not yet made an impact, smoking is on the increase, and tobacco companies market their products without restriction.

❦ To cease smoking is the easiest thing I ever did. I ought to know because I've done it a thousand times. ❦

Mark Twain, US author.

sperm or spermatozoon
The male gamete or sex cell. Each sperm cell has a head capsule containing a nucleus, a middle portion containing mitochondria (which provide energy), and a long tail (flagellum). Sperm cells are produced in the testes (see **testis**). From there they pass through the sperm ducts via the seminal vesicles and the **prostate gland**, which

produce fluids called **semen** that give the sperm cells energy and keep them moving after they leave the body. Hundreds of millions of sperm cells are contained in only a small amount of semen. The human sperm is 0.005 mm/ 0.0002 in long and can survive inside the female for 2–9 days.

sphincter
Ring of muscle, such as is found at various points in the alimentary canal, that contracts and relaxes to open and close the canal and control the movement of food. The pyloric sphincter, at the base of the **stomach**, controls the release of the gastric contents into the duodenum. After release the sphincter contracts, closing off the stomach.
See also: *digestive system.*

spina bifida
Congenital defect in which part of the spinal cord and its membranes are exposed due to incomplete development of the spine (vertebral column). It is a neural tube defect. Spina bifida, usually present in the lower back, varies in

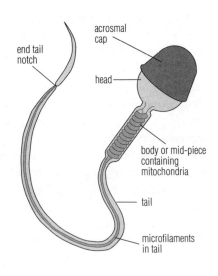

acrosmal cap

end tail notch

head

body or mid-piece containing mitochondria

tail

microfilaments in tail

sperm *Only a single sperm is needed to fertilize an egg, or ovum. Yet up to 500 million may start the journey towards the egg. Once a sperm has fertilized an egg, the egg's wall cannot be penetrated by other sperm. The unsuccessful sperm die after about three days.*

It has been established that adequate quantities of folic acid in the mother's diet can prevent the condition. The UK government now officially advises women who are planning to a pregnancy, or who are already pregnant, to increase their intake of folic acid to 400 micrograms daily.

severity. The most seriously affected babies may be paralyzed below the waist. There is also a risk of mental retardation and death from **hydrocephalus**, which is often associated. Surgery is performed to close the spinal lesion shortly after birth but this does not usually cure the disabilities caused by the condition. Spina bifida can be diagnosed prenatally.

spinal cord
Major component of the **central nervous system**. It consists of bundles of nerves enveloped in three layers of membrane (the meninges) and is bathed in cerebrospinal fluid. The spinal cord is encased and protected by the vertebral column, lying within the vertebral canal formed by the posterior arches of successive **vertebrae**. The spinal cord extends from the bottom of the **skull**, where it is continuous with the lowest part of the brainstem, to about waist level. It consists of nerve cell bodies (grey matter) and their myelinated processes or nerve fibres (white matter). Paired spinal nerves arise from the cord at each vertebra. Each is a mixed nerve, consisting of both sensory and motor nerve fibres.

spleen
Organ which is part of the reticuloendothelial system concerned with fighting infection and which helps to process lymphocytes (type of **white blood cells**). It also regulates the number of **red blood cells** in circulation by destroying old cells and stores iron. It is situated on the left side of the body, behind the stomach.

sprain
Injury to a ligament resulting in over-stretching. The most commonly sprained joint is the ankle. Immediate symptoms are pain and loss of power in the joint, followed by swelling. Swelling can be minimized by applying cold water immediately. After the joint has swollen, however, heat should be used to ease the pain. The sprained part should be well bandaged and rested. It may take months to recover fully.

sputum
Saliva together with **mucus** coughed up from the airways.

Squint or strabismus
Common condition in which one **eye** deviates in any direction. A squint may be convergent (with the bad eye turned inwards), divergent (outwards) or, in rare cases, vertical. A convergent squint is also called cross-eye. There are two types of squint: paralytic, arising from disease or damage involving the extraocular muscles or their nerve supply; and nonparalytic, which may be inherited or due to some refractive error within the eye. Nonparalytic (or concomitant) squint is the typical condition seen in small children. It is treated by corrective glasses, exercises for the eye muscles, or surgery.

stammer
Disorder affecting the fluency of speech in which certain sounds, syllables, or words may be repeated while other sounds are prolonged or blocked. Stammering may be associated with grimacing or gesturing and its severity may increase at times of stress. A stammer usually begins in childhood and affects boys more than girls. It can be treated by teaching appropriate control of breathing and measured sound production.

sterility
Inability to reproduce. It may be due to infertility or it may be induced (**sterilization**).

sterilization
Any surgical operation to terminate the possibility of reproduction. In women, this is normally achieved by sealing or tying off the **Fallopian tubes** (tubal ligation) so that **fertilization** can no longer take place. In men, the transmission of **sperm** is blocked by **vasectomy**.

sternum or breastbone
The large flat bone, 15–20 cm/5.9–7.8 in long in the adult, at the front of the chest, joined to the ribs. It gives protection to the **heart** and **lungs**. The sternum can be felt beneath the skin throughout its whole length, from the root of the neck into the abdominal wall. It has three parts: the manubrium, body, and xiphoid process which

are united by **cartilage**. The joint between the manubrium and body, the sternal angle, can be felt opposite the second ribs.

stethoscope

Instrument used to ascertain the condition of the **heart** and **lungs** by listening to their action. It consists of two earpieces connected by flexible tubes to a small plate that is placed against the body. It was invented in 1819 in France by René Théophile Hyacinthe Laënnec.

stomach

The first cavity in the **digestive system**. It is a bag of muscle situated just below the diaphragm. Food enters it from the **oesophagus**, is digested by the acid and enzymes secreted by the stomach lining and then passes into the duodenum.

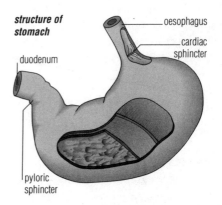

structure of stomach

oesophagus
cardiac sphincter
duodenum
pyloric sphincter

stroke

(Also known as cerebrovascular accident, or apoplexy). Interruption of the blood supply to part of the brain due to a sudden bleed in the brain (cerebral **haemorrhage**) or **embolism**, or **thrombosis**. Strokes vary in severity from producing almost no symptoms to proving rapidly fatal. In between are those (often recurring) that leave a wide range of impaired function, depending on the size and location of the event. Strokes

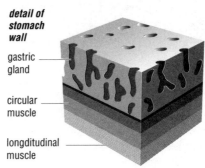

detail of stomach wall

gastric gland
circular muscle
longditudinal muscle

stomach *The human stomach can hold about 1.5 l/2.6 pt of liquid. The digestive juices are acidic enough to dissolve metal. To avoid damage, the cells of the stomach lining are replaced quickly – 500,000 cells are replaced every minute, and the whole stomach lining every three days.*

involving the right side of the brain, for example, produce weakness of the left side of the body. Some affect speech. Around 80% of strokes are ischaemic strokes, caused by a blood clot blocking an artery transporting blood to the brain. Transient ischaemic attacks (**TIAs**), or 'mini-strokes', with effects lasting only briefly (less than 24 hours), require investigation to try to forestall the possibility of a subsequent full-blown stroke. The disease of the arteries that predisposes to stroke is **atherosclerosis**. **High blood pressure** (**hypertension**) is also a precipitating factor. Strokes can sometimes be prevented by surgery (as in the case of some **aneurysms**) or medication. The **clot-buster** drug tPA, if administered within three hours of a stroke, can cut the number of stroke victims experiencing lasting disability by 50%.

stye
Bacterial infection of a gland at the base of an eyelash. It causes inflammation and the formation of pus.

sunstroke
Heatstroke caused by excessive exposure to the sun.

suppository
Drug or other therapeutic preparation manufactured in solid form for insertion into the **vagina** or rectum (see **digestive system**).

symptom
Any change or manifestation in the body suggestive of disease as perceived by the sufferer. In strict usage, symptoms are events or changes reported by the patient; signs are noted by the doctor during the patient's examination.

syndrome
A set of signs and symptoms that always occur together, thus characterizing a particular condition or disorder.

syphilis
Sexually transmitted disease or **venereal disease** caused by the spi-

ral-shaped bacterium (spiro-
chete) *Treponema pallidum.*
Untreated, it runs its course
in three stages over many
years, often starting with a
painless hard sore, or chan-
cre, developing within a
month on the area of infec-

Undergarments with a mercury coating were sometimes worn as a precautionary measure to protect the wearer against syphilis in 17th-century Italy.

tion (usually the **genitalia**). The second stage, months later, is a rash with arthritis, **hepatitis,** and/or **meningitis**. The third stage, years later, leads eventually to **paralysis**, blindness, insanity, and death. With widespread availability of **antibiotics**, syphilis is now increas-ingly treatable in the industrialized world, at least to the extent that the final stage of the disease is rare. The risk remains that the disease may go undiagnosed or that it may be transmitted by a pregnant woman to her **fetus**.

tapeworm

Any of various parasitic flatworms of the class *Cestoda*. They lack digestive and sense organs, can reach 15 m/50 ft in length, and attach themselves to the host's intestines by means of hooks and suckers. Tapeworms are made up of hundreds of individual segments, each of which develops into a functional hermaphroditic reproductive unit capable of producing numerous eggs. The larvae of tapeworms usually reach humans in imperfectly cooked meat or fish, causing **anaemia** and intestinal disorders.

Tay–Sachs disease

Inherited disorder, due to a defective **gene**, causing an enzyme deficiency that leads to blindness, retardation, and death in infancy. It is most common in people of Eastern European Jewish descent.

tendon or sinew

Cord of very strong, fibrous connective tissue that joins **muscle** to **bone**. Tendons are largely composed of bundles of fibres made of the protein collagen, and because of their inelasticity are very efficient at transforming muscle power into movement. Tendons are attached at one end to the sarcolemma or connective tissue around muscle fibres and at the other end to the periosteum, the connective tissue surrounding bone. Tendons have a relatively poor blood supply and heal slowly if they are torn.

tennis elbow

Painful condition of the elbow due to over-use of the forearm muscles. It is a form of tendinitis.

testis

The organ (part of the **genitalia**) that produces **sperm** in males. The paired testes (or testicles) descend from the body cavity during development, to hang outside the abdomen in a scrotal sac. The testes also secrete the male sex hormone androgen.

testosterone

Hormone secreted chiefly by the **testes** but also by the **ovaries** and the cortex (outer part) of the adrenal glands. It promotes the development of secondary sexual characteristics in males. Like other sex hormones, testosterone is a steroid.

tetanus or lockjaw

Acute disease caused by the **toxin** of the bacillus *Clostridium tetani*, which usually enters the body through a wound. The bacterium is chiefly found in richly manured soil. Untreated, in seven to ten days tetanus produces muscular spasm and rigidity of the jaw spreading to other parts of the body, **convulsions,** and death. There is a **vaccine** and the disease may be treatable with tetanus antitoxin and **antibiotics**.

thalassaemia or Cooley's anaemia

Any of a group of chronic hereditary blood disorders that are widespread in the Mediterranean countries, Africa, the Far East, and the Middle East. They are characterized by an abnormality of the **red blood cells** and bone marrow, with enlargement of the **spleen**. The **genes** responsible are carried by about 100 million people worldwide. The diseases can be diagnosed prenatally.

thorax

The part of the body containing the **heart** and **lungs** and protected by the ribcage. The thorax is separated from the abdomen by the muscular diaphragm. The thoracic inlet contains the oesophagus (gullet) and **trachea** (windpipe), and those arteries and veins leading from and to the heart through the neck, together with certain nerves. The thoracic outlet is filled by the diaphragm. The intercostal spaces between adjacent ribs are sealed by three layers of intercostal muscles. During inspiration these muscles lift the ribs and the diaphragm flattens, causing an increase in volume of the thorax. The lungs expand to fill this extra space, drawing in air. During expiration the relaxation of the intercostal muscles and diaphragm, combined with the elastic recoil of the lungs, forces air out of the lungs.

thrombosis
Condition in which a blood clot forms in a vein or artery, causing loss of circulation to the area served by the vessel. If it breaks away, it often travels to the lungs, causing pulmonary **embolism**.

Thrombosis in veins of the legs is often seen in association with phlebitis, and in arteries with the fatty deposits known as atheroma. Thrombosis increases the risk of **heart attack** and **stroke**. It is treated by surgery and/or anticoagulant drugs.

thrush
Infection usually of the mouth (particularly in infants), but also sometimes of the vagina, caused by a yeastlike fungus (*Candida albicans*). It is seen as white patches on the **mucous membranes**. Thrush, also known as candidiasis, may be caused by **antibiotics** removing natural antifungal agents from the body. It is treated with a further antibiotic.

thyroid
Endocrine gland situated in the neck in front of the **trachea**. It secretes several **hormones**, principally thyroxine, an iodine-containing hormone that stimulates growth, **metabolism**, and other functions of the body. The thyroid gland may be thought of as the regulator gland of the body's metabolic rate. If it is overactive, as in **hyperthyroidism**, the sufferer feels hot and sweaty, has an increased heart rate, diarrhoea, and weight loss. Conversely, an underactive thyroid leads to myxoedema, a condition characterized by sensitivity to cold, constipation, and weight gain. In infants, an underactive thyroid leads to cretinism, a form of mental retardation.

TIA
Abbreviation for transient ischaemic attack. Popularly known as a 'mini-**stroke**', it is a sudden loss of function in one part of the brain.

Symptoms may include: double vision or temporary loss of vision, speech difficulties, vomiting, loss of sensation and perhaps movement on one side of the body, dizziness, unsteadiness, loss of memory, and momentary collapse; loss of consciousness is rare. Symptoms usually reach a peak within seconds and last for minutes or perhaps hours. Recovery is complete but TIAs tend to recur.

tinnitus
Constant buzzing or ringing in the **ears**. The phenomenon may originate from prolonged exposure to noisy conditions (drilling, machinery, or loud music) or from damage to or disease of the middle or inner ear. The victim may become overwhelmed by the relentless noise in the head.

tonsils
Masses of lymphoid tissue situated at the back of the mouth and throat (palatine tonsils) and on the rear surface of the tongue (lingual tonsils). The tonsils contain many lymphocytes, (type of **white blood cells**) and are part of the body's defence system against infection. The adenoids are sometimes called pharyngeal tonsils.

tooth
One of a set of hard, bonelike structures in the mouth, used for biting and chewing food. The first set (20 milk teeth) appear from age six months to two and a half years. The permanent dentition replaces these from the sixth year onwards, the wisdom teeth (third molars) sometimes not appearing until the age of 25 or 30. Adults have 32 teeth:
- two incisors
- one canine (eye tooth)
- two premolars
- three molars on each side of each jaw.

Each tooth consists of an enamel coat (hardened calcium deposits), dentine (a thick, bonelike layer), and an inner pulp cavity, housing nerves and blood vessels. Teeth have roots surrounded by

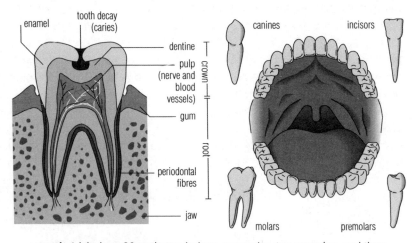

tooth *Adults have 32 teeth: two incisors, one canine, two premolars, and three molars on each side of each jaw. Each tooth has three parts: crown, neck, and root. The crown consists of a dense layer of mineral, the enamel, surrounding hard dentine with a soft centre, the pulp.*

cementum, which fuses them into their sockets in the jawbones. The neck of the tooth is covered by the gum, while the enamel-covered crown protrudes above the gum line. The chief diseases of teeth are misplacements resulting from defect or disturbance of the tooth-germs before birth, eruption out of their proper places, and caries (decay).

> ❢ To lose a lover or even a husband or two during the course of one's life can be vexing. But to lose ones teeth is a catastrophe. ❣
>
> **Hugh Wheeler**, *A Little Night Music.*

toxic shock syndrome

Rare condition marked by rapid onset of fever, vomiting, and low **blood pressure,** sometimes leading to death. It is caused by a toxin of the bacterium *Staphylococcus aureus*, normally harmlessly present in the body. It is seen most often in young women using tampons during **menstruation**.

toxin
Any **poison** produced by another living organism (usually a **bacterium**) that can damage the living body. Toxins are broken down by enzyme action, mainly in the **liver**.

trachea or windpipe
Tube that forms an airway and runs from the larynx to the upper part of the chest. It is strong and flexible, and reinforced by rings of **cartilage**. In the upper chest, the trachea branches into two tubes: the left and right bronchi, which enter the **lungs**.

tranquillizer
Common name for any drug for reducing **anxiety** or tension (anxiolytic), such as benzodiazepines, barbiturates, antidepressants, and beta-blockers. The use of drugs to control anxiety is becoming much less popular because many of them are capable of inducing dependence.

transfusion
Intravenous delivery of blood or blood products (**plasma**, **red blood cells**) into a patient's circulation to make up for deficiencies due to disease, injury, or

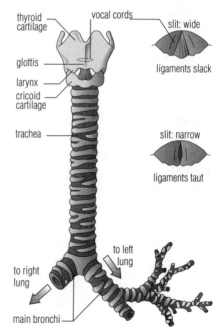

trachea *The human trachea, or windpipe. The larynx, or voice box, lies at the entrance to the trachea. The two vocal cords are membranes that normally remain open and still. When they are drawn together, the passage of air makes them vibrate and produce sounds.*

surgical intervention. Cross-matching is carried out to ensure the patient receives the right **blood group**. Because of worries about blood-borne disease, there is a growing interest in autologous transfusion with units of the patient's own blood 'donated' over the weeks before an operation.

Blood transfusion, first successfully pioneered in humans in 1818, remained a high-risk procedure until the discovery of blood groups by Austrian-born immunologist Karl **Landsteiner** in 1900, which indicated the need for compatibility of donated blood.

transplant

The transfer of a tissue or organ from one human being to another or from one part of the body to another (skin grafting). In most organ transplants, the operation is for life-saving purposes, although the immune system tends to reject foreign tissue. Careful matching and immunosuppressive drugs must be used, but these are not always successful. Corneal grafting, which may restore sight to a diseased or damaged eye, was pioneered in 1905, and is the oldest successful human transplant procedure. Of the internal organs, **kidneys** were first transplanted successfully in the early 1950s and remain most in demand. Modern transplantation also encompasses the **heart**, **lungs**, **liver**, pancreatic tissue, small bowel, **bone**, and bone-marrow.

Most transplant material is taken from cadaver donors, usually those suffering death of the brainstem, or from frozen tissue banks. In rare cases, kidneys, corneas, and part of the liver may be obtained from living donors. Besides the shortage of donated material, the main problem facing transplant surgeons is rejection of the donated organ by the recipient's body.

> ❛The human body is the only machine for which there are no spare parts.❜
>
> **Hermann M Biggs.**

trauma

In **psychiatry**, a painful emotional experience or shock with lasting psychic consequences; in medicine, any physical damage or injury.
 In psychiatric terms a trauma may have long-lasting effects during which an insignificant event triggers the original distress. A person then may have difficulties in normal life, such as in establishing relationships or sleeping. This is known as post-traumatic stress disorder. It can be treated by psychotherapy.

tuberculosis (TB)

Formerly known as consumption. Infectious disease caused by the bacillus *Mycobacterium tuberculosis*. It takes several forms, of which pulmonary tuberculosis is by far the most common. A **vaccine**, BCG, was developed around 1920 and the first anti-tuberculosis drug, streptomycin, in 1944. The bacterium is mostly kept in check by the body's immune system; about 5% of those infected develop the disease. In pulmonary TB, a patch of inflammation develops in the lung, with formation of an **abscess**. Often, this heals spontaneously, leaving only scar tissue. The dangers are of rapid spread through both lungs or the development of miliary tuberculosis (spreading in the bloodstream to other sites) or tuberculous **meningitis**.

- In 1999 there were 8 million new cases of TB and 2 million deaths.
- Only 5% of cases are in developed countries.
- Worldwide there are 16 million people with TB and 2 billion (a third of the global population) are infected with *M. tuberculosis*.
- Over the last 15 years there has been a sharp resurgence in countries where the disease was in decline.
- Treatment of patients with a combination of anti-TB medicines for 6–8 months usually produces a cure rate of 80%.
- However, the last decade has seen the spread of drug-resistant strains of the TB bacterium. Many strains are now resistant to the two frontline drugs, isoniazid and rifampicin, and some are multidrug resistant (MDR).

- In the US, a clear link between TB and HIV, the virus which causes **AIDS**, has been established.

tumour
Overproduction of cells in a specific area of the body, often leading to a swelling or lump. Tumours are classified as benign or malignant (see **cancer**). Benign tumours grow more slowly, do not invade surrounding tissues, do not spread to other parts of the body, and do not usually recur after removal. However, benign tumours can be dangerous in areas such as the **brain**. The most familiar types of benign tumour are **warts** on the skin. In some cases, there is no sharp dividing line between benign and malignant tumours.

twin
One of two offspring produced from a single pregnancy. Twins may be genetically identical (monozygotic), having been formed from a single fertilized egg that splits into two cells, both of which became implanted. Nonidentical (fraternal or dizygotic) twins are formed when two eggs are fertilized at the same time.

ulcer

Any persistent breach in a body surface (**skin** or **mucous membrane**). It may be caused by infection, irritation, or **tumour** and is often inflamed. Common ulcers include aphthous (mouth), gastric (stomach), duodenal, decubitus ulcers (**pressure sores**), and those complicating varicose veins. Treatment of ulcers depends on the site. Drugs are the first line of attack against peptic ulcers (those in the digestive tract),

The presence of *H. pylori* in the stomach can be detected by a breathtest.

though surgery may become necessary. Bleeding stomach ulcers can be repaired without an operation by the use of **endoscopy**: a flexible fibre-optic tube is passed into the stomach and under direct vision fine instruments are used to repair the tissues. Stomach ulcers are linked to the **bacteria** *Helicobacter pylori* found in the stomachs of 60% of adults in the West by the time they are 60. One in six infected with the bacterium develops ulcers. They are twice as common in those with blood type O, which may be because *H. pylori* attaches itself to the stomach lining by a string of sugar found only in that blood group.

> 6 I don't have ulcers; I give them. 9
>
> **Harry Cohn**, US film producer.

ULCER TREATMENT

- Headless bedbugs were aplied to ulcers in the 16th century, and crushed bedbugs were still believed to be effective in treatng ulcers in 18th-century China.
- It was not until this century that positive evidence was found of the antibacterial properties of insect haemolymph.

ultrasound scanning or ultrasonography

The use of ultrasonic pressure waves to create a diagnostic image. It is a safe, noninvasive technique that often eliminates the need for exploratory surgery. The sound waves transmitted through the body are absorbed and reflected to different degrees by different body tissues.

umbilical cord

Connection between the **embryo** and the **placenta**. It has one vein and two arteries, transporting oxygen and nutrients to the developing **fetus** and removing waste products. At birth, the connection between the baby and the placenta is no longer necessary. The umbilical cord drops off or is severed, leaving a scar called the navel.

urinary system

System of organs that removes nitrogenous waste products and

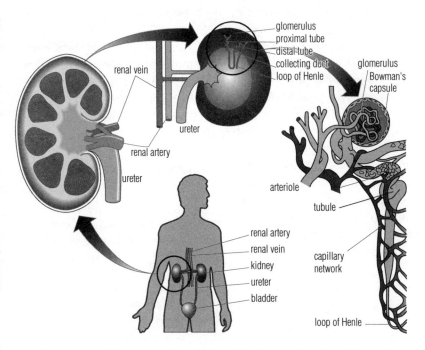

urinary system *The human urinary system. At the bottom, the complete system in outline; on the left, the arrangement of blood vessels connected to the kidney; at the top right, a detail of the network of vessels within a kidney.*

excess water from the body. It consists of a pair of **kidneys**, which produce urine; ureters, which drain the kidneys; and a bladder that stores the urine before its discharge. Urine is expelled through the urethra.

urticaria or nettle rash or hives

Irritant skin condition characterized by itching, burning, stinging, and the spontaneous appearance of raised patches of skin. Treatment is usually by **antihistamines** or steroids taken orally or applied as lotions. Its causes are varied and include **allergy** and stress.

uterus

Hollow muscular organ of females, located between the bladder and rectum, and connected to the **Fallopian tubes** above and the **vagina** below. The **embryo** develops within the uterus and is attached to it after implantation via the **placenta** and **umbilical cord**. The lining of the uterus changes during the **menstrual cycle**. The outer wall of the uterus is composed of smooth **muscle** capable of powerful contractions (induced by **hormones**) during childbirth.

vaccine
Any preparation of modified pathogens (**viruses** or **bacteria**) that is introduced into the body, usually either orally or by injection, to produce **immunity** against a particular disease.

> 6 Vaccination is the medical sacrament corresponding to baptism. 9
>
> **Samuel Butler**, British writer.

vagina
The lower part of the reproductive tract in females, linking the **uterus** to the exterior. It admits the penis during sexual intercourse and is the birth canal down which the baby passes during delivery.

varicose veins or varicosis
Condition where the veins become swollen and twisted. The veins of the legs are most often affected; other vulnerable sites include the rectum (**piles**) and **testes**. Some people have an inherited tendency to varicose veins and the condition often appears in pregnant women, but obstructed blood flow is the direct cause. They may cause a dull ache or may be the site for thrombosis, infection, or ulcers. The affected veins can be injected with a substance that causes them to shrink or surgery may be needed.

vasectomy
Male **sterilization** – an operation to cut and tie the ducts that carry sperm from the testes to the penis. Vasectomy does not affect sexual performance, but the semen produced at ejaculation no longer contains sperm.

vein

Any vessel that carries blood from the body to the heart. Veins contain valves that prevent the blood from running back when moving against gravity. They carry blood at low pressure so their walls are thinner than those of arteries. They always carry deoxygenated blood, with the exception of the pulmonary veins, leading from the lungs to the heart, which carry newly oxygenated blood.

venereal disease (VD)

(VD). Any disease mainly transmitted by sexual contact, although commonly the term is used specifically for **gonorrhoea** and **syphilis**, both occurring worldwide, and chancroid ('soft sore') and lymphogranuloma venerum, seen mostly in the tropics. The term **sexually transmitted disease** (STD) is more often used to encompass a growing list of conditions passed on primarily, but not exclusively, by sexual contact.

ventilator

Machine that assists or maintains **breathing** when a patient is unable to breathe normally due to illness or injury. There are two modes of ventilation in medical use: positive pressure and negative pressure. The more widely used is the positive pressure ventilator, sometimes popularly known as a 'life-support machine'. With this, air is blown through an endotracheal tube down the back of the throat to inflate the **lungs**; the air is exhaled when the pressure from the ventilator is released. Usually this mode of ventilation is only needed for a short time.

The iron lung is an example of a negative pressure ventilator. The patient lies encased in it, with only the head exposed. A vacuum is created inside the chamber, causing the chest wall to expand and drawing air into the lungs; as the vacuum is released the chest wall subsides, expelling air from the lungs. This mode of assisted ventilation is suitable for people with chronic breathing difficulties, including some **polio** victims.

verruca

Growth on the skin; see **wart**.

vertebra
An irregularly shaped bone that forms part of the vertebral column (**spine**). Children have 33 vertebrae, 5 of which fuse in adulthood to form the sacrum and 4 to form the coccyx. There are 7 cervical vertebrae in the neck, 12 thoracic vertebrae in the thorax with the ribs attached and 5 lumbar vertebrae in the lower back.
See also: *skeleton.*

vertigo
Dizziness; a whirling sensation accompanied by a loss of any feeling of contact with the ground. It may be due to temporary disturbance of the sense of balance (as in spinning for too long on one spot), psychological reasons, disease such as labyrinthitis, or intoxication.
See also: *ear.*

Virchow, Rudolf Ludwig Carl (1821–1902)
German pathologist and founder of cellular pathology. In his book *Die Cellulare Pathologie/Cellular Pathology* (1858), he proposed that disease is the cell's response to altered and abnormal conditions within the body. It is not due to sudden changes but to slow processes in which normal cells give rise to abnormal ones. Virchow was the first to describe **leukaemia**.

virus
Infectious particle consisting of a core of nucleic acid (**DNA** or **RNA**) enclosed in a protein shell. Viruses are able to function and reproduce only if they can invade a living **cell** to use the cell's system to replicate themselves. In the process they may disrupt or alter the host cell's own DNA. The healthy human body reacts by producing an antiviral protein, interferon, which prevents the infection spreading to adjacent cells.

Many viruses mutate continuously so that the host's body has little chance of developing permanent resistance; others transfer between species, with the new host similarly unable to develop resistance. The viruses that cause **AIDS** and Lassa fever (occuring in Central West Africa) are both thought to have 'jumped' to humans from other mammalian hosts.

Among other diseases caused by viruses are **chickenpox, herpes,**

influenza, rabies, and yellow fever (a disease of the tropics and subtropics). Viruses are also implicated in the development of some **cancers.**

Antiviral drugs are difficult to develop because viruses replicate by using the genetic machinery of host cells so that drugs tend to affect the host cell as well as the virus. Some viruses have developed resistance to the few antiviral drugs available.

vitamin
Any of various chemically unrelated organic compounds that are necessary in small quantities for the normal functioning of the human body. Many act as coenzymes, small molecules that enable enzymes to function effectively. Vitamins must be supplied by the diet because the body cannot make them. They are normally present in adequate amounts in a balanced diet but vitamin supplements are widely available. Deficiency of a vitamin may lead to a metabolic disorder ('deficiency disease'), which can be remedied by sufficient intake of the vitamin. They are generally classified as water-soluble (B and C) or fat-soluble (A, D, E, and K).

Scurvy (the result of vitamin C deficiency) was observed at least 3,500 years ago, and sailors from the 1600s were given fresh sprouting cereals or citrus-fruit juices to prevent or cure it. The concept of scurvy as a deficiency disease, however, caused by the absence of a specific substance, emerged later. In the 1890s a Dutch doctor, Christiaan Eijkman, discovered that he could cure hens suffering from a condition like beriberi (caused by a deficiency of thiamine or vitamin B1) by feeding them on whole-grain, rather than polished, rice. In 1912 Casimir Funk, a Polish-born biochemist, had proposed the existence of what he called 'vitamines' (vital amines), but it was not fully established until about 1915 that several deficiency diseases were preventable and curable by extracts from certain foods.

vocal cords
The paired folds, ridges, or cords of tissue within the larynx (forming part of the air passage to the lungs). Air constricted between the folds or membranes makes them vibrate, producing sounds. Muscles in the larynx change the pitch of the sounds produced, by adjusting the tension of the vocal cords.

See also: *laringitis.*

wart

Protuberance composed of a local overgrowth of skin. The common wart (*Verruca vulgaris*) is due to a virus infection. It usually disappears spontaneously within two years, but can be treated with peeling applications, burning away (cautery), freezing (cryosurgery), or laser treatment.

whiplash injury

Damage to the neck vertebrae and their attachments caused by a sudden backward jerk of the head and neck. It is most often seen in vehicle occupants as a result of the rapid deceleration experienced in a crash.

white blood cell or leucocyte

One of a number of different cells that play a part in the body's defences and give immunity against disease. Some (neutrophils and macrophages) engulf invading micro-organisms, others kill infected cells, while lymphocytes produce more specific immune responses. White blood cells are colourless, with clear or granulated cytoplasm, and are capable of independent amoeboid movement. They occur in the blood, lymph, and elsewhere in the body's tissues.

Unlike **red blood cells**, they possess a nucleus. Human blood contains about 11,000 leucocytes to the cubic millimetre – about one to every 500 red cells.

White blood cell numbers may be reduced (leucopenia) by starvation, pernicious anaemia, and certain infections, such as typhoid and malaria. An increase in their numbers (leucocytosis) is a reaction to normal events such as digestion, exertion, and pregnancy, and to abnormal ones such as loss of blood, cancer, and most infections.

whooping cough or pertussis

Acute infectious disease, seen mainly in children, caused by colonization of the air passages by the bacterium *Bordetella pertussis*. There may be catarrh, mild fever, and loss of appetite, but the main symptom is violent coughing, associated with the sharp intake of breath that is the characteristic 'whoop', and often followed by vomiting and severe nose bleeds. The cough may persist for weeks.

Although debilitating, the disease is seldom serious in older children, but infants are at risk both from the illness itself and from susceptibility to other conditions, such as pneumonia. Immunization lessens the incidence and severity of the disease. The whole cell (or 'killed') vaccine has been replaced by an acellular version which has fewer side effects than its predecessor.

X-ray

Band of electromagnetic radiation. Applications of X-rays make use of their short wavelength or their penetrating power (as in medical X-rays of internal body tissues). X-rays are dangerous and can cause **cancer**. X-rays with short wavelengths pass through most body tissues, although dense areas such as bone prevent their passage, showing up as white areas on X-ray photographs. The X-rays used in radiotherapy have very short wavelengths that penetrate tissues deeply and destroy them. X-rays were discovered by German experimental physicist Wilhelm **Röntgen** in 1895 and formerly called rontgen rays.

yellow fever

Acute tropical viral disease, prevalent in the Caribbean area, Brazil, and on the west coast of Africa. The yellow fever virus is an arbovirus transmitted by mosquitoes. Its symptoms include a high fever, headache, joint and muscle pains, vomiting, and yellowish skin (jaundice, possibly leading to liver failure); the heart and kidneys may also be affected. The mortality rate is 25%, with 91% of all cases occurring in Africa. Before the arrival of Europeans, yellow fever was not a problem because indigenous people had built up an immunity. The disease was brought under control after the discovery that it is carried by the mosquito *Ae{uml}des aegypti*. The first effective **vaccines** were produced by Max Theiler (1899–1972) of South Africa, for which he was awarded the 1951 Nobel Prize for Medicine.

The World Health Organization (WHO) estimates there are about 200,000 cases of yellow fever each year in Africa, with 30,000 deaths (1993).

zoonosis

Any infectious disease that can be transmitted to humans by other vertebrate animals. Probably the most feared example is **rabies**. The transmitted micro-organism sometimes causes disease only in the human host, leaving the animal host unaffected.

Appendix

Major drugs derived from plants

Many of these plants are poisonous and if swallowed can cause serious illness or unconsciousness. They should only be used if administered by a medically trained professional.

Plant	Drug	Use
Amazonian liana	curare	muscle relaxant
Annual mugwort	artemisinin	antimalarial
Autumn crocus	colchicine	antitumour agent
Camphor tree camphor	rubefacient	used in insect repellents and medicinal inhalants and liniments
Coca cocaine	local anaesthetic	
Common thyme thymol	antifungal	
Deadly nightshade (belladonna)	atropine	anticholinergic
Dog button (nux-vomica)	strychnine	central nervous system stimulant
Ergot fungus	ergotamine	analgesic
Foxglove	digitoxin, digitalis	cardiotonic
Indian snakeroot	reserpine	antihypertensive
Meadowsweet	salicylate	analgesic
Mexican yam	diosgenin	birth control pill
Mint, peppermint	menthol	rubefacient
Opium poppy	codeine, morphine	analgesic (codeine is also antitussive)
Pacific yew taxol	antitumour agent	
Recured thornapple	scopolamine	sedative
Rosy periwinkle	vincristine, vinblastine	antileukaemia
Tea, coffee, and kola nuts	caffeine	central nervous system stimulant
Velvet bean	L-dopa	antiparkinsonian
White willow	salicylic acid	topical analgesic
Yellow cinchona	quinine antimalarial,	antipyretic

Human body: composition

Chemical element or substance Body weight (%)

Pure elements

Oxygen	65
Carbon	18
Hydrogen	10
Nitrogen	3
Calcium	2
Phosphorus	1.1
Potassium	0.35
Sulphur	0.25
Sodium	0.15
Chlorine	0.15

Magnesium, iron, manganese, copper, iodine, cobalt, zinc traces

Water and solid matter

Water	60–80
Total solid material	20–40
Organic molecules	
Protein	15–20
Lipid	3–20
Carbohydrate	1–15
Other	0–1

Western Medicine: Key Events

c. 400 BC	Hippocrates recognizes that disease had natural causes.
c. AD 200	Galen consolidates the work of the Alexandrian doctors.
1543	Andreas Vesalius gives the first accurate account of the human body.
1628	William Harvey discovers the circulation of the blood.
1768	John Hunter begins the foundation of experimental and surgical pathology.
1785	Digitalis is used to treat heart disease; the active ingredient is isolated in 1904.
1798	Edward Jenner publishes his work on vaccination.
1877	Patrick Manson studies animal carriers of infectious diseases.
1882	Robert Koch isolates the bacillus responsible for tuberculosis.
1884	Edwin Klebs isolates the diphtheria bacillus.
1885	Louis Pasteur produces a vaccine against rabies.
1890	Joseph Lister demonstrates antiseptic surgery.
1895	Wilhelm Röntgen discovers X-rays.
1897	Martinus Beijerinck discovers viruses.
1899	Felix Hoffman develops aspirin; Sigmund Freud founds psychiatry.
1900	Karl Landsteiner identifies the first three blood groups, later designated A, B, and O.

1910	Paul Ehrlich develops the first specific antibacterial agent, Salvarsan, a cure for syphilis.
1922	Insulin is first used to treat diabetes.
1928	Alexander Fleming discovers penicillin.
1932	Gerhard Domagk discovers the first antibacterial sulphonamide drug, Prontosil.
1937	Electro-convulsive therapy (ECT) is developed.
1940s	Lithium treatment for manic-depressive illness is developed.
1950s	Antidepressant drugs and beta-blockers for heart disease are developed. Manipulation of the molecules of synthetic chemicals becomes the main source of new drugs. Peter Medawar studies the body's tolerance of transplanted organs and skin grafts.
1950	Proof of a link between cigarette smoking and lung cancer is established.
1953	Francis Crick and James Watson announce the structure of DNA. Jonas Salk develops a vaccine against polio.
1958	Ian Donald pioneers diagnostic ultrasound.
1960s	A new generation of minor tranquillizers called benzodiazepines is developed.
1967	Christiaan Barnard performs the first human heart transplant operation.
1971	Viroids, disease-causing organisms even smaller than viruses, are isolated outside the living body.
1972	The CAT scan, pioneered by Godfrey Hounsfield, is first used to image the human brain.
1975	César Milstein develops monoclonal antibodies.
1978	World's first 'test-tube baby' is born in the UK.
1980s	AIDS (acquired immuno-deficiency syndrome) is first recognized in the USA. Barbara McClintock's discovery of the transposable gene is recognized.
1980	The World Health Organization reports the eradication of smallpox.
1983	The virus responsible for AIDS, now known as human immunodeficiency virus (HIV), is identified by Luc Montagnier at the Institut Pasteur, Paris; Robert Gallo at the National Cancer Institute, Maryland, USA discovers the virus independently in 1984.
1984	The first vaccine against leprosy is developed.
1987	The world's longest-surviving heart-transplant patient dies in France, 18 years after his operation.
1989	Grafts of fetal brain tissue are first used to treat Parkinson's disease.
1990	Gene for maleness is discovered by UK researchers.
1991	First successful use of gene therapy (to treat severe combined immune deficiency) is reported in the USA.
1993	First trials of gene therapy against cystic fibrosis take place in the USA.
1996	An Australian man, Ben Dent, is the first person to end his life by legally sanctioned euthanasia.
1990s	A strain of typhoid fever that is resistant to all known antibiotics emerges in the late 1990s.
1999	The UK Department of Health announces that all pregnant women in England and Wales will be offered an HIV test. HIV transmission to newborns can be cut from 15 to 2 % by antiviral therapy, Caesarean section delivery, and bottle feeding.

Bones of the Human Body

Bone		Number
Cranium (skull)	Occipital	1
	Parietal: 1 pair	2
	Sphenoid	1
	Ethmoid	1
	Inferior nasal conchae	2
	Frontal: 1 pair, fused	1
	Nasal: 1 pair	2
	Lacrimal: 1 pair	2
	Temporal: 1 pair	2
	Maxilla: 1 pair, fused	1
	Zygomatic: 1 pair	2
	Vomer	1
	Palatine: 1 pair	2
	Mandible (jawbone): 1 pair, fused	1
	Total	21
Ear	Malleus (hammer)	1
	Incus (anvil)	1
	Stapes (stirrups)	1
	Total (2 x 3)	6
Vertebral column (spine)	Cervical vertebrae	7
	Thoracic vertebrae	12
	Lumbar vertebrae	5
	Sacral vertebrae: 5, fused to form the sacrum	1
	Coccygeal vertebrae: between 3 and 5, fused to form the coccyx	1
	Total	26
Ribs	Ribs, "true": 7 pairs	14
	Ribs, "false": 5 pairs, of which 2 pairs are floating	10
	Total	24
Sternum (breastbone)	Manubrium, sternebrae ("body"), and xiphisternum	
	Total	3
Throat	Hyoid	1
	Total	1
Pectoral girdle	Clavicle: 1 pair (collarbone)	2
	Scapula (including coracoid): 1 pair (shoulder-blade)	2
	Total	4
Upper extremity (each arm)		
Forearm	humerus	1
	radius	1
	ulna	1

Bone		Number
Carpus (wrist)	scaphoid	1
	lunate	1
	triquetral	1
	pisiform	1
	trapezium	1
	trapezoid	1
	capitate	1
	hamate	1
	metacarpals	5
Phalanges (fingers)	first digit	2
	second digit	3
	third digit	3
	fourth digit	3
	fifth digit	3
	Total (2 x 30)	60
Pelvic girdle	Ilium, ischium, and pubis (combined): 1 pair of hip bones,	
	innominate	2
	Total	2
Lower extremity (each leg)		
Leg	femur (thighbone)	1
	tibia (shinbone)	1
	fibula	1
	patella (kneecap)	1
Tarsus (ankle)	talus	1
	calcaneus	1
	navicular	1
	cuneiform, medial	1
	cuneiform, intermediate	1
	cuneiform, lateral	1
	cuboid	1
	metatarsals (foot bones)	5
Phalanges (toes)	first digit	2
	second digit	3
	third digit	3
	fourth digit	3
	fifth digit	3
	Total (2 x 30)	60
TOTAL		207

Immunization: Key Events

AD 23–79   Pliny the Elder suggests using liver from mad dogs as protection against rabies.
1500s   Asian physicians immunize against smallpox using the crusts from pustules. This is only partially successful.
1720s   Lady Mary Wortley Montagu introduces smallpox immunization into Europe from Turkey.
1796   British physician Edward Jenner develops a safe smallpox vaccine using the cowpox virus.
1853   Vaccination against smallpox is made compulsory in Britain.
1885   French microbiologist Louis Pasteur develops a vaccine for rabies.
1894–1904   German immunologist Emil von Behring and Japanese bacteriologist Kitasato Shibasaburo successfully test vaccines for diphtheria and tetanus.
1896   A E Wright develops typhoid vaccine.
1914   Tetanus vaccine becomes available on a large scale.
1920s   Tuberculosis vaccine produced.
1937   South African-born US microbiologist Max Theiler develops vaccine 17-D, still the main form of protection against yellow fever.
1949   Whooping cough vaccine licensed.
1952   US microbiologist Jonas Salk develops the first successful vaccine for poliomyelitis.
1960s   Measles and rubella vaccines produced.
1961   The oral vaccine for poliomyelitis, developed by Russian-born virologist Albert Sabin, becomes widely available.
1967   The World Health Organization (WHO) begins its global campaign against smallpox.
1970s   Vaccines produced for meningococcal diseases and chickenpox. The WHO begins constructing its "cold chain" to ensure adequate transport and refrigeration for vaccines, which can take up to two years to reach their target in a developing country.
1974   WHO launches the Expanded Programme on Immunization, as fewer than 5% of children in developing countries are currently immunized.
1978   Pulmonary disease vaccine is developed.
1980s   Vaccine for hepatitis B, and a combination vaccine for measles, mumps, and rubella (MMR) becomes available.
1980   Smallpox virtually eradicated.
1984   Leprosy vaccine developed.
1989–1990   More than 100 children die when a measles epidemic sweeps through several large cities in the USA, highlighting the failure of the immunization programme. Three-quarters of the 45,000 children affected have not been vaccinated.
1990   Vaccine introduced for 'Hemophilus influenzae', a cause of meningitis.
1991   WHO estimates 80% of the world's children are immunized against diphtheria, whooping cough, tetanus, measles, polio, and tuberculosis. A US survey of nine major cities finds that less than half of school-age children have been fully vaccinated against infectious diseases by their second birthday.
1994   Fear of a measles epidemic in the UK leads to a vaccination programme for all children aged 5–16.
1995   First human trials of a vaccine administered by eating genetically engineered potatoes.
1996   Heat-sensitive chemical monitors used on polio vaccine containers from January. If the monitor changes colour health workers will know that high temperatures have destroyed

1998
the vaccine. A vaccine for salmonella for use in poultry is approved in Australia. Controversy arises over the use of the combined MMR vaccine owing to the claims of a UK paediatrician that there is a slight risk of immunized children developing autism in later life. This risk did not exist when the vaccinations were given as three separate shots at different times. In India, the government authorizes the sale of the world's first leprosy vaccine; in 1998 there are an estimated 1.5 million cases of leprosy of which 60% are in India. The vaccine is only effective for 6–12 months.

AIDS: Key Dates

1977
Two men in New York are diagnosed as having the rare cancer Kaposi's sarcoma. They are thought to be the first victims of AIDS.

1979
The Center for Disease Control in Atlanta, Georgia, reports the first cases of the disease later known as AIDS.

1981
The Center for Disease Control in Atlanta, Georgia, first conclusively identifies AIDS; doctors realize they have previously seen similar cases among drug users and homosexuals.

1983
US medical researcher Robert Gallo at the US National Cancer Institute, Maryland, and French medical researcher, Luc Montagnier, at the Pasteur Institute in Paris, isolate the virus thought to cause AIDS; it becomes known as HIV (human immunodeficiency virus).

20 March 1987
The AIDS treatment drug AZT is given approval by the US Food and Drug Administration. Treatment costs $10,000 per year per patient. The treatment does not cure the disease but it does relieve some symptoms and extend victims' lives.

31 December 1994
The number of AIDS cases worldwide exceeds 1 million for the first time, when the World Health Organization (WHO) announces that there are 1,025,073 officially reported AIDS cases.

1995
US researchers estimate that HIV reproduces at a rate of a billion viruses a day, even in otherwise healthy individuals, but is held at bay by the immune system producing enough white blood cells to destroy them. Gradually the virus mutates so much that the immune system is overwhelmed and the victim develops AIDS.

9 May 1996
Scientists discover a protein, "fusin", which allows the HIV virus to fuse with a human immune system cell's outer membrane and inject genetic material. Its presence is necessary for the AIDS virus to enter the cell.

September 1996
The first three protease inhibitors are approved by the US Food and Drug Administration (FDA). Protease inhibitors are a new type of antiretroviral (a drug that stops the reproduction of HIV in the body).

January 1997
WHO estimates that 22.6 million men, women, and children have to date been infected by HIV, the virus responsible for causing AIDS. Approximately 42% of adult sufferers are female, with the proportion of women infected steadily increasing.

February 1997
The Centers for Disease Control and Prevention in Atlanta, Georgia, report that deaths among people with AIDS declined 13% during the first six months of 1996 over the same period the year before.

8 May 1997
US AIDS researcher David Ho and colleagues show how aggressive treatment of HIV-1 infection with a cocktail of three antiviral drugs can drive the virus to below the limits of conventional clinical detection within eight weeks.

9 February 1998 David Ho reports the discovery of the AIDS virus in a 1959 blood sample and suggests that a transfer of the virus from ape to human occurred in the late 1940s or early 1950s.

March 1998 According to a new study, a protein found in the urine of pregnant women could stop the reproduction of HIV, the virus that causes AIDS. The protein is known as human chorionic gonadotropin, or hcg. It also boosts the immune system and, because it is produced by the human body, is nontoxic and has very few side effects.

30 June 1998 Doctors report for the first time the ominous spread of a strain of the AIDS virus that is resistant to protease inhibitors, the medicines that have revolutionized care of the disease.

October 1998 Children born today in 29 sub-Saharan African nations face a life expectancy of just 47 years because of the toll the AIDS pandemic is taking on the region, according to a UN population report.

December 1998 Researchers report they have identified an inherited gene variation that in some patients causes an HIV infection to accelerate rapidly to AIDS. The identification of all the gene variations involved in both the rapid acceleration of HIV and in the slow progress of the disease would help in the design and testing of vaccines.

January 1999 WHO estimates that 33.4 million adults and children are living with AIDS at the end of 1998. Deaths due to HIV/AIDS in 1998 totalled 2.5 million, while the cumulative number of deaths reached 13.9 million.

January 1999 Researchers say they have conclusive evidence that the HIV virus has spread on at least three separate occasions from chimpanzees to humans in Africa. Chimps, which probably carried the virus for hundreds of thousands of years, apparently do not become ill from it. Understanding why, say AIDS experts, could help in a search for a cure and in the development of a vaccine.

February 1999 Thailand gives permission to the US company VaxGen Inc. to begin advance testing of an AIDS vaccine on about 2,500 people. The California-based company has already done preliminary trials of AIDSVAX vaccine on up to 90 Thai drug users.

About 30 possible AIDS vaccines are in development, but AIDSVAX is the first to undergo massive testing to determine if it prevents AIDS infection.

February 1999 The first trial of an AIDS vaccine in Africa begins in a group of Ugandans considered at low risk of contracting the disease.

16 March 1999 US scientists report they have isolated an enzyme present in tears, which they believe has a powerful anti-HIV effect.

19 April 1999 The AIDS epidemic in South Africa reaches alarming new levels, with 10% of the population now infected with HIV. A national survey confirmed that the country has one of the highest rates of infection in the world.

21 April 1999 Hundreds of demonstrators rally in Washington, DC, to protest at policies which they say protect drug companies but make AIDS drugs too expensive for people in Africa.

April 1999 Scientists at Yerkes Regional Primate Center in Georgia, USA, announce that a "safe" HIV vaccine has been successfully tested on monkeys. The vaccine, that uses harmless parts of HIV, protected monkeys from extremely virulent strains of the virus for at least 62 weeks.

12 May 1999 AIDS is now the leading cause of death in Africa, overtaking malaria as the continent's main killer disease, according to the UN.

1 June 1999 A new easier-to-take AIDS drug—Efavirenz—which has been hailed as "a major advance in the treatment of HIV infection", is granted a licence for sale in the EU. It was approved in the USA the previous summer.

16 July 1999 Researchers in the USA and Uganda say they have identified a cheap and effective drug—called Nevirapine—which could control the spread of AIDS. The drug could prevent up to 400,000 children each year being born with the disease.

23 September 1999 Drug-resistant strains of HIV are on the increase, with as many as 3.8% of newly infected Americans failing to respond to a variety of different treatments, according to a study carried out by the AIDS Research Center at Rockerfeller University in New York.

November 1999 More than 50 million people are now infected with the HIV virus, according to UN and WHO estimates. More than 16 million have died from AIDS-related illnesses.

7 March 2000 Virologists at Thomas Jefferson University in Philadelphia say they have developed an HIV vaccine using a weakened rabies virus to carry a piece of the HIV virus safely into the cells of laboratory mice. The cells respond by creating immune system antibodies to attack the fragment, thus increasing their long-term capacity to fight off the HIV virus.

31 March 2000 A combination of drugs introduced in 1997 to treat HIV is shown to have dramatically increased the lifespan of patients, according to a comprehensive study carried out in Europe. The study shows that the drug combination known as Haart (highly-active antiretroviral therapy) is responsible for an overall decline of 64% in the risk of dying from AIDS within 10 years of developing the virus.

30 April 2000 The US government formally designates AIDS as a threat to international security and orders a major reassessment of its efforts against the disease. The Clinton administration acts after intelligence reports warn that the AIDS epidemic could trigger wars and genocide and undermine democratic governments, particularly in Africa.

2 May 2000 More than four out of every five deaths in Rwanda are now AIDS-related, according to government officials.
The figure—which covers the preceding three months—was given at an international conference on AIDS by Rwanda's health minister.

9 July 2000 The world's 13th conference on AIDS commences in South Africa. Botswanan President Festus Mogae warns that AIDS is causing a national crisis. Over a third of Botswanan adults is infected with HIV. Thabo Mbeki, president of South Africa, who had controversially claimed there was no link between HIV and AIDS, insists that poverty, not the virus, is the real killer.

Common Allergies

Allergy is extremely widespread and now affects 1 in 4 of the UK population at some time during their lifetime.

Each year the numbers are increasing by 5%.

The most common allergy in the UK is hay fever which can occur at any age and in early 2000 affected 20% of all allergy sufferers.

This table is meant as a guide only. Always consult a doctor if you have any concerns or doubts.

Allergy	Cause	Symptoms/comments
Pollen allergy (hay fever)	mainly grass and tree pollen	allergic rhinitis (running eyes and nose, sneezing, nasal congestion), eczema, urticaria (nettlerash or hives), and asthma; asthma symptoms range from mild to moderate or severe and can be life-threatening; people with the disease suffer "attacks", or acute episodes, when the air passages in their lungs narrow and breathing becomes difficult; affects more than 3 million people in the UK, including one in every seven school children and one in every 25 adults
Dust-mite allergy	enzymes in the faeces of mites in house dust, feathers, pillows, and mattresses	symptoms as above, though they tend to be primarily respiratory in nature; affects about 5% of the UK population (1999)
Pet allergy	allergens in the pet's saliva, urine, or skin flakes, carried on its fur	symptoms as above
Mould allergy	spores from moulds growing in damp living spaces and on hay and cereal grain	symptoms as above, though they tend to be primarily respiratory in nature; moulds can be found both indoors and outdoors and allergies are often associated with pollen allergies
Insect bite or sting allergy	proteins in the venom	severe and prolonged swelling at the site of the sting, pain, and—in extreme cases—anaphylactic shock (respiratory difficulties, a rapid fall in blood pressure, and collapse, followed by loss of consciousness and even death); sufferers may also experience abdominal pain, vomiting, and diarrhoea
Food allergy	most commonly to proteins in dairy foods, eggs, peanuts, true nuts, wheat and soya products, and shellfish, or to chemicals such as monosodium glutamate, tartrazine, sulphur	eczema, urticaria, asthma, itching around the mouth, vomiting, diarrhoea, and—in extreme cases—anaphylactic shock (see above); the most visible signs of the onset of anaphylactic shock resulting from food allergies are often swelling and rashes on the lips and tongue; food allergy is often confused with food intolerance, which is not

Allergy	Cause	Symptoms/comments
	dioxide, and sodium benzoate in food additives	caused by the body's immune response but by its inability to digest a particular food (for example, lactose intolerance) or by adverse reactions to drug-like chemicals such as caffeine in coffee and amines in chocolate and cheese; peanut allergies affect about 0.5% of the UK population
Drug allergy	most commonly to the antibiotics penicillin and tetracycline, sulfonamides, streptomycin, and local anaesthetics such as novocaine and lidocaine	signs of an allergic reaction include fever, urticaria, itchy nose, throat or ears, and flushed skin; symptoms of a stronger reaction may include coughing, swelling—especially of the eyes or tongue, and cyanosis, a bluish tint of the skin; anaphylactic shock can be triggered by drugs like morphine or the dye injected prior to X-raying; the horse serum used in the makeup of some vaccines can also cause anaphylactic shock
Latex allergy	latex, the processed form of the milky sap derived from natural rubber trees, used mainly in gloves and many other medical products such as IV tubing and catheters, as well as in condoms, shoe soles, and swimming goggles	early symptoms include eczema, urticaria, and flushing, often followed by itching, congestion, eye irritation, wheezing, asthma, and progression into anaphylaxis; while direct skin contact is a problem, the allergen can also be inhaled—this occurs primarily when the gloves are removed and the protein which has combined with the powder inside the glove becomes airborne; those allergic to the following foods may also be sensitive to latex: avocados, bananas, potatoes, tomatoes, hazelnuts, chestnuts, kiwi, and papayas

Vitamins

Vitamin	Name	Main dietary sources	Established benefit	Deficiency symptoms
A	retinol	dairy products, egg yolk, liver; also formed in body from β-carotene, a pigment present in some leafy vegetables	aids growth; prevents night blindness and xerophthalmia (a common cause of blindness among children in developing countries); helps keep the skin and mucous membranes resistant to infection	night blindness; rough skin; impaired bone growth
B_1	thiamin	germ and bran of seeds and grains, yeast	essential for carbohydrate metabolism and health of nervous system	beriberi; Korsakov's syndrome
B_2	riboflavin	eggs, liver, milk, poultry, broccoli, mushrooms	involved in energy metabolism; protects skin, mouth, eyes, eyelids, mucous membranes	inflammation of tongue and lips; sores in corners of the mouth

Vitamin	Name	Main dietary sources	Established benefit	Deficiency symptoms
B_6 kidney	pyridoxine/ pantothenic acid/biotin	meat, poultry, fish, fruits, nuts, whole grains, leafy vegetables, yeast extract	important in the regulation of the central nervous system and in protein metabolism; helps prevent anaemia, skin lesions, nerve damage	dermatitis; neurological problems; stones
B_{12}	cyanoco-balamin	liver, meat, fish, eggs, dairy products, soybeans	involved in synthesis of nucleic acids, maintenance of myelin sheath around nerve fibres; efficient use of folic acid	anaemia; neurological disturbance
	folic acid	green leafy vegetables, liver, peanuts; cooking and processing can cause serious losses in food	involved in synthesis of nucleic acids; helps protect against cervical dysplasia (precancerous changes in the cells of the uterine cervix)	megaloblastic anaemia
	nicotinic acid (or niacin)	meat, yeast extract, some cereals; also formed in the body from the amino acid tryptophan	maintains the health of the skin, tongue, and digestive system	pellagra
C	ascorbic acid	citrus fruits, green vegetables, tomatoes, potatoes; losses occur during storage and cooking	prevents scurvy, loss of teeth; fights haemorrhage; important in synthesis of collagen (constituent of connective tissue); aids in resistance to some types of virus and bacterial infections	scurvy
D children;	calciferol, chole-calciferol	liver, fish oil, dairy products, eggs; also produced when skin is exposed to sunlight	promotes growth and mineralization of bone	rickets in osteomalacia in adults
E	tocopherol	vegetable oils, eggs, butter, some cereals, nuts	prevents damage to cell membranes	anaemia
K	phytom-enadione, mena-quinone	green vegetables, cereals, fruits, meat, dairy products	essential for blood clotting	haemorrhagic problems

Nobel Prize for Physiology or Medicine

Year	Winner(s)[1]	Awarded for
1901	Emil von Behring (Germany)	discovery that the body produces antitoxins, and development of serum therapy for diseases such as diphtheria
1902	Ronald Ross (UK)	work on the role of the 'Anopheles' mosquito in transmitting malaria
1903	Niels Finsen (Denmark)	discovery of the use of ultraviolet light to treat skin diseases
1904	Ivan Pavlov (Russia)	discovery of the physiology of digestion
1905	Robert Koch (Germany)	investigations and discoveries in relation to tuberculosis
1906	Camillo Golgi (Italy) and Santiago Ramón y Cajal (Spain)	discovery of the fine structure of the nervous system
1907	Charles Laveran (France)	discovery that certain protozoa can cause disease
1908	Ilya Mechnikov (Russia) and Paul Ehrlich (Germany)	work on immunity
1909	Emil Kocher (Switzerland)	work on the physiology, pathology, and surgery of the thyroid gland
1910	Albrecht Kossel (Germany)	study of cell proteins and nucleic acids
1911	Allvar Gullstrand (Sweden)	work on the refraction of light through the different components of the eye
1912	Alexis Carrel (France)	work on the techniques for connecting severed blood vessels and transplanting organs
1913	Charles Richet (France)	work on allergic responses
1914	Robert Bárány (Austria-Hungary)	work on the physiology and pathology of the equilibrium organs of the inner ear
1915	no award	
1916	no award	
1917	no award	
1918	no award	
1919	Jules Bordet (Belgium)	work on immunity
1920	August Krogh (Denmark)	discovery of the mechanism regulating the dilation and constriction of blood capillaries
1921	no award	
1922	Archibald Hill (UK)	work in the production of heat in contracting muscle
	Otto Meyerhof (Germany)	work in the relationship between oxygen consumption and metabolism of lactic acid in muscle
1923	Frederick Banting (Canada) and John Macleod (UK)	discovery and isolation of the hormone insulin
1924	Willem Einthoven (Netherlands)	invention of the electrocardiograph
1925	no award	
1926	Johannes Fibiger (Denmark)	discovery of a parasite 'Spiroptera carcinoma' that causes cancer
1927	Julius Wagner-Jauregg (Austria)	use of induced malarial fever to treat paralysis caused by mental deterioration

Year	Winner(s)[1]	Awarded for
1928	Charles Nicolle (France)	work on the role of the body louse in transmitting typhus
1929	Christiaan Eijkman (Netherlands)	discovery of a cure for beriberi, a vitamin-deficiency disease
	Frederick Hopkins (UK)	discovery of trace substances, now known as vitamins, that stimulate growth
1930	Karl Landsteiner (USA)	discovery of human blood groups
1931	Otto Warburg (Germany)	discovery of respiratory enzymes that enable cells to process oxygen
1932	Charles Sherrington (UK) and Edgar Adrian (UK)	discovery of function of neurons (nerve cells)
1933	Thomas Morgan (USA)	work on the role of chromosomes in heredity
1934	George Whipple (USA), George Minot (USA), and William Murphy (USA)	work on treatment of pernicious anaemia by increasing the amount of liver in the diet
1935	Hans Spemann (Germany)	organizer effect in embryonic development
1936	Henry Dale (UK) and Otto Loewi (Germany)	chemical transmission of nerve impulses
1937	Albert Szent-Györgyi (Hungary)	investigation of biological oxidation processes and of the action of ascorbic acid (vitamin C)
1938	Corneille Heymans (Belgium)	mechanisms regulating respiration
1939	Gerhard Domagk (Germany)	discovery of the first antibacterial sulphonamide drug
1940	no award	
1941	no award	
1942	no award	
1943	Henrik Dam (Denmark)	discovery of vitamin K
	Edward Doisy (USA)	chemical nature of vitamin K
1944	Joseph Erlanger (USA) and Herbert Gasser (USA)	transmission of impulses by nerve fibres
1945	Alexander Fleming (UK)	discovery of the bactericidal effect of penicillin
	Ernst Chain (UK) and Howard Florey (Australia)	isolation of penicillin and its development as an antibiotic drug
1946	Hermann Muller (USA)	discovery that X-ray irradiation can cause mutation
1947	Carl Cori (USA) and Gerty Cori (USA)	production and breakdown of glycogen (animal starch)
	Bernardo Houssay (Argentina)	function of the pituitary gland in sugar metabolism
1948	Paul Müller (Switzerland)	discovery of the first synthetic contact insecticide DDT
1949	Walter Hess (Switzerland)	mapping areas of the midbrain that control the activities of certain body organs
	Antonio Egas Moniz (Portugal)	therapeutic value of prefrontal leucotomy in certain psychoses
1950	Edward Kendall (USA), Tadeus Reichstein (Switzerland), and Philip Hench (USA)	structure and biological effects of hormones of the adrenal cortex
1951	Max Theiler (South Africa)	discovery of a vaccine against yellow fever
1952	Selman Waksman (USA)	discovery of streptomycin, the first antibiotic effective against tuberculosis

Year	Winner(s)[1]	Awarded for
1953	Hans Krebs (UK)	discovery of the Krebs cycle
	Fritz Lipmann (USA)	discovery of coenzyme A, a nonprotein compound that acts in conjunction with enzymes to catalyse metabolic reactions leading up to the Krebs cycle
1954	John Enders (USA), Thomas Weller (USA), and Frederick Robbins (USA)	cultivation of the polio virus in the laboratory
1955	Hugo Theorell (Sweden)	work on the nature and action of oxidation enzymes
1956	André Cournand (USA), Werner Forssmann (West Germany), and Dickinson Richards (USA)	work on the technique for passing a catheter into the heart for diagnostic purposes
1957	Daniel Bovet (Italy)	discovery of synthetic drugs used as muscle relaxants in anaesthesia
1958	George Beadle (USA) and Edward Tatum (USA)	discovery that genes regulate precise chemical effects
	Joshua Lederberg (USA)	work on genetic recombination and the organization of bacterial genetic material
1959	Severo Ochoa (USA) and Arthur Kornberg (USA)	discovery of enzymes that catalyse the formation of RNA (ribonucleic acid) and DNA (deoxyribonucleic acid)
1960	Macfarlane Burnet (Australia) and Peter Medawar (UK)	acquired immunological tolerance of transplanted tissues
1961	Georg von Békésy (USA)	investigations into the mechanism of hearing within the cochlea of the inner ear
1962	Francis Crick (UK), James Watson (USA), and Maurice Wilkins (UK)	discovery of the double-helical structure of DNA and of the significance of this structure in the replication and transfer of genetic information
1963	John Eccles (Australia), Alan Hodgkin (UK), and Andrew Huxley (UK)	ionic mechanisms involved in the communication or inhibition of impulses across neuron (nerve cell) membranes
1964	Konrad Bloch (USA) and Feodor Lynen (West Germany)	work on the cholesterol and fatty-acid metabolism
1965	François Jacob (France), André Lwoff (France), and Jacques Monod (France)	genetic control of enzyme and virus synthesis
1966	Peyton Rous (USA)	discovery of tumour-inducing viruses
	Charles Huggins (USA)	hormonal treatment of prostatic cancer
1967	Ragnar Granit (Sweden), Haldan Hartline (USA), and George Wald (USA)	physiology and chemistry of vision
1968	Robert Holley (USA), Har Gobind Khorana (USA), and Marshall Nirenberg (USA)	interpretation of genetic code and its function in protein synthesis
1969	Max Delbrück (USA), Alfred Hershey (USA), and Salvador Luria (USA)	replication mechanism and genetic structure of viruses
1970	Bernard Katz (UK), Ulf von Euler (Sweden), and Julius Axelrod (USA)	work on the storage, release, and inactivation of neurotransmitters

Year	Winner(s)[1]	Awarded for
1971	Earl Sutherland (USA)	discovery of cyclic AMP, a chemical messenger that plays a role in the action of many hormones
1972	Gerald Edelman (USA) and Rodney Porter (UK)	work on the chemical structure of antibodies
1973	Karl von Frisch (Austria), Konrad Lorenz (Austria), and Nikolaas Tinbergen (UK)	work in animal behaviour patterns
1974	Albert Claude (USA), Christian de Duve (Belgium), and George Palade (USA)	work in structural and functional organization of the cell
1975	David Baltimore (USA), Renato Dulbecco (USA), and Howard Temin (USA)	work on interactions between tumour-inducing viruses and the genetic material of the cell
1976	Baruch Blumberg (USA) and Carleton Gajdusek (USA)	new mechanisms for the origin and transmission of infectious diseases
1977	Roger Guillemin (USA) and Andrew Schally (USA)	discovery of hormones produced by the hypothalamus region of the brain
	Rosalyn Yalow (USA)	radioimmunoassay techniques by which minute quantities of hormone may be detected
1978	Werner Arber (Switzerland), Daniel Nathans (USA), and Hamilton Smith (USA)	discovery of restriction enzymes and their application to molecular genetics
1979	Allan Cormack (USA) and Godfrey Hounsfield (UK)	development of the computed axial tomography (CAT) scan
1980	Baruj Benacerraf (USA), Jean Dausset (France), and George Snell (USA)	work on genetically determined structures on the cell surface that regulate immunological reactions
1981	Roger Sperry (USA)	functional specialization of the brain's cerebral hemispheres
	David Hubel (USA) and Torsten Wiesel (Sweden)	work on visual perception
1982	Sune Bergström (Sweden), Bengt Samuelsson (Sweden), and John Vane (UK)	discovery of prostaglandins and related biologically active substances
1983	Barbara McClintock (USA)	discovery of mobile genetic elements
1984	Niels Jerne (Denmark-UK), Georges Köhler (West Germany), and César Milstein (Argentina)	work on immunity and discovery of a technique for producing highly specific, monoclonal antibodies
1985	Michael Brown (USA) and Joseph L Goldstein (USA)	work on the regulation of cholesterol metabolism
1986	Stanley Cohen (USA) and Rita Levi-Montalcini (USA-Italy)	discovery of factors that promote the growth of nerve and epidermal cells
1987	Susumu Tonegawa (Japan)	work on the process by which genes alter to produce a range of different antibodies
1988	James Black (UK), Gertrude Elion (USA), and George Hitchings (USA)	work on the principles governing the design of new drug treatment

Year	Winner(s)[1]	Awarded for
1989	Michael Bishop (USA) and Harold Varmus (USA)	discovery of oncogenes, genes carried by viruses that can trigger cancerous growth in normal cells
1990	Joseph Murray (USA) and Donnall Thomas (USA)	pioneering work in organ and cell transplants
1991	Erwin Neher (Germany) and Bert Sakmann (Germany)	discovery of how gatelike structures (ion channels) regulate the flow of ions into and out of cells
1992	Edmond Fischer (USA) and Edwin Krebs (USA)	isolating and describing the action of the enzyme responsible for reversible protein phosphorylation, a major biological control mechanism
1993	Phillip Sharp (USA) and Richard Roberts (UK)	discovery of split genes (genes interrupted by nonsense segments of DNA)
1994	Alfred Gilman (USA) and Martin Rodbell (USA)	discovery of a family of proteins (G-proteins) that translate messages—in the form of hormones or other chemical signals—into action inside cells
1995	Edward Lewis (USA), Eric Wieschaus (USA), and Christiane Nüsslein-Volhard (Germany)	discovery of genes which control the early stages of the body's development
1996	Peter Doherty (Australia) and Rolf Zinkernagel (Switzerland)	discovery of how the immune system recognizes virus-infected cells
1997	Stanley Prusiner (USA)	discoveries, including the "prion" theory, that could lead to new treatments of dementia-related diseases, including Alzheimer's and Parkinson's diseases
1998	Robert Furchgott (USA), Ferid Murad (USA), and Louis Ignarro (USA)	discovery that nitric oxide (NO) acts as a key chemical messenger between cells
1999	Günter Blobel (USA)	discovery that proteins have intrinsic signals that govern their transport and localization in the cell

[1] Nationality given is the citizenship of recipient at the time award was made.

BSE: Key Dates

1985   An epidemic of bovine spongiform encephalopathy (BSE or "mad cow disease") is reported in beef cattle in Britain; it is later traced to cattle feed containing sheep carcasses infected with scrapie.

November 1986   BSE first formally identified by Central Veterinary Laboratory.

15 May 1990   Home-produced beef is banned in UK schools and hospitals as a result of concern about bovine spongiform encephalopathy.

25 March 1996   The European Union bans the export of British beef abroad following anxiety over the potential for transmission of the BSE infection to humans as CJD (Creutzfeldt-Jakob disease).

1 April   The agriculture minister Douglas Hogg proposes a scheme to eradicate BSE in Britain

1996	and get the export ban on British beef lifted; 4.6 million cattle over 6 years old would be culled.
1 August 1996	The UK Central Veterinary Laboratory publishes a report indicating that BSE can be transmitted from cow to calf.
2 October 1997	UK scientists Moira Bruce and, independently, John Collinge, and their colleagues show that the new variant form of the brain-wasting CJD is the same disease as bovine spongiform encephalopathy in cows.
3 December 1997	Agriculture Secretary Jack Cunningham announces that the government will ban the sale of beef on the bone to help prevent the transmission of BSE to humans.
November 1998	The government announces £120 million emergency aid package for Britain's farmers to compensate for the BSE crisis.
	Later that month, the European Union partially lifts the ban on the export of British beef pending slaughterhouse inspections.
4 March 1998	EU veterinarians approve the removal of the ban of British beef exports from Northern Ireland. The decision has to be ratified by the EC.
9 March 1998	Public inquiry into the origin and spread of BSE and its human equivalent, CJD, opens in London.
16 March 1998	EU agricultural ministers vote to allow beef from herds in Northern Ireland to be sold abroad again. Northern Ireland becomes the first part of the UK to see the two-year beef ban lifted because it has a computer-based system to keep track of cattle.
17 March 1998	The Agriculture Minister, Jack Cunningham, says the final bill for combating the BSE outbreak would top £4 billion.
December	Phase One (fact finding) hearings of the BSE Inquiry are completed; its report is scheduled to be delivered to Ministers June 1999; this is later postponed to March 2000.
January 1999	Scientists announce they have developed a test for CJD which could show the extent of the disease in the population. The test involves taking tissue from the tonsils and can be conducted on living people. The test also suggests CJD may be more infectious than thought and could be spread through routine surgery.
March 1999	The critical moment when Creutzfeld-Jakob disease or BSE strikes the brain is captured in a test tube for the first time. The breakthrough, by the Medical Research Council's Prion Unit, is a major step forward for the future development of new diagnostic tests and possibly even effective treatments of the disease.
April 1999	The number of people known to have died of the human form of BSE rises to 40. The total number of people who died from CJD in 1998 stands at 16, a sharp increase on previous years.
	Evidence that the ban was flouted and that contaminated cattle reached the food chain until 1996, means some people may have caught the disease in the 1990s. The government's scientific researchers call for more research to find out if BSE has passed to sheep which were given the same feed as infected cattle.
2000	Analysis of tissue from thousands of removed appendices held in hospitals failed to detect signs of CJD in the British population.